an introduction to
ESSENTIAL OILS

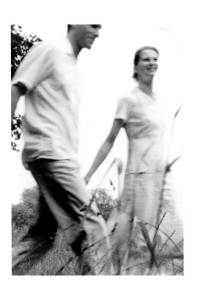

p

an introduction to
ESSENTIAL OILS

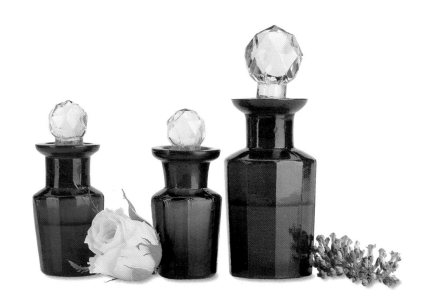

Sara Rose

This is a Parragon Publishing book
This edition published in 2002

Parragon Publishing
Queen Street House
4 Queen Street
Bath, BA1 1HE, UK

This book was created by
THE BRIDGEWATER BOOK COMPANY

A CIP catalogue record for this book is
available from the British Library

ISBN 0-75258 880-X

Printed in China

Contents

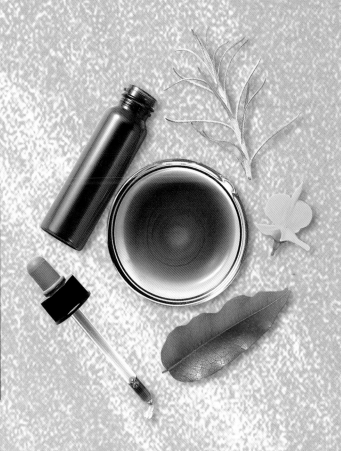

Introduction

Essential oils are complex chemical substances extracted from plant material, which can be used to promote good health and well-being, and to treat illness. Each oil is made up of a combination of hundreds of different components that give the oil its individual scent, dominant characteristics, and gentle but effective healing properties. Essential oils are now commonly used in industry, and have been incorporated into a wide range of commercial products, from air fresheners to washing-up liquid.

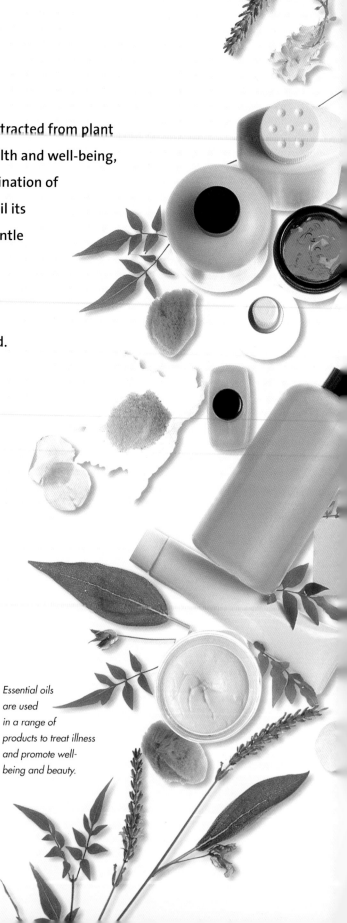

E ssential oils have been used throughout history to treat illness and promote well-being and beauty. Although it was not always known how they worked, we now understand that many of these oils have specific properties that enable them to counter infection and disease.

The use of essential oils today, generally inhaled or applied to the skin, is one of the fastest growing areas of complementary medicine. It is an excellent example of a holistic approach to health, in which the mind, body, and spirit are treated as a whole and the body's natural self-healing processes are stimulated.

The first section of this book is an introduction to essential oils, how they work and how to use them. An extensive photographic catalog of the most popular essential oils follows, with a description of their main properties and characteristics. The third part describes how the oils can be used to treat a range of common ailments. The final part of the book contains a brief glossary, and a list of useful addresses, along with a comprehensive index.

Essential oils are used in a range of products to treat illness and promote well-being and beauty.

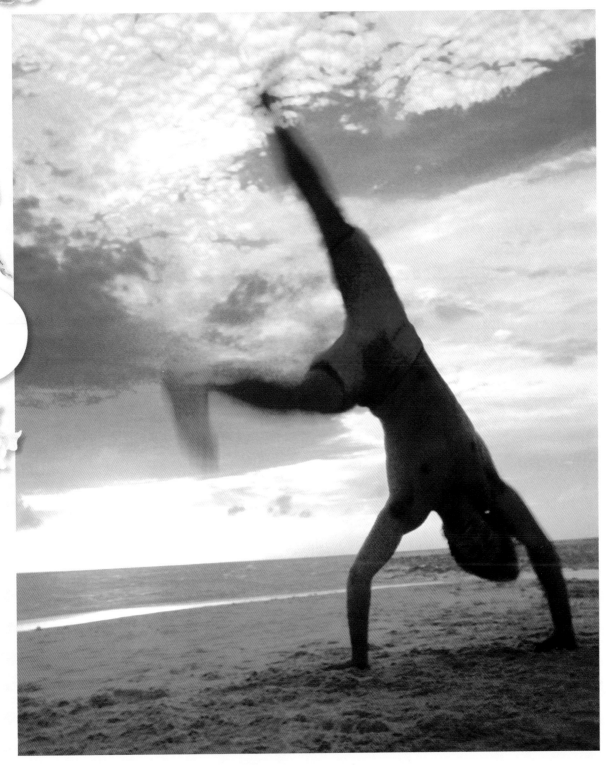

*Essential oils are used in a holistic approach to
health, in which the mind, body, and spirit
are seen as connected and the body is
encouraged to heal itself.*

What are **essential oils?**

Many plants contain tiny pockets of aromatic oils—natural chemicals that attract pollinating insects and defend against pest damage and fungi. These oils have many health-giving properties.

Essential oils, which give a plant its characteristic smell and flavor, may be contained in any part of it, from the roots to the flowers. Oils are extracted from bushes, flowers, trees, and shrubs all over the world and each has a unique chemical composition. This section describes the history of their use, how they work and their health benefits, methods of extraction and how to prepare them, safety measures, and the most common ways of using essential oils.

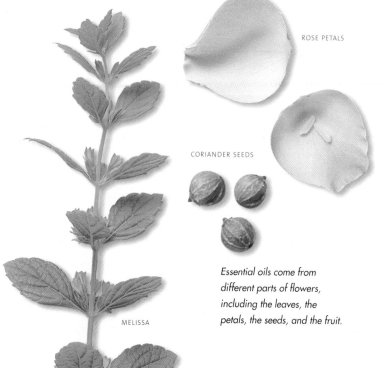

LIME

ROSE PETALS

CORIANDER SEEDS

MELISSA

Essential oils come from different parts of flowers, including the leaves, the petals, the seeds, and the fruit.

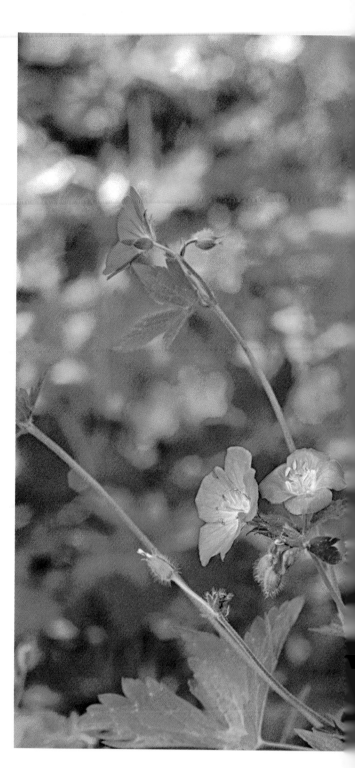

Geranium flowers produce a remedy that calms, balances, and soothes the nervous system.

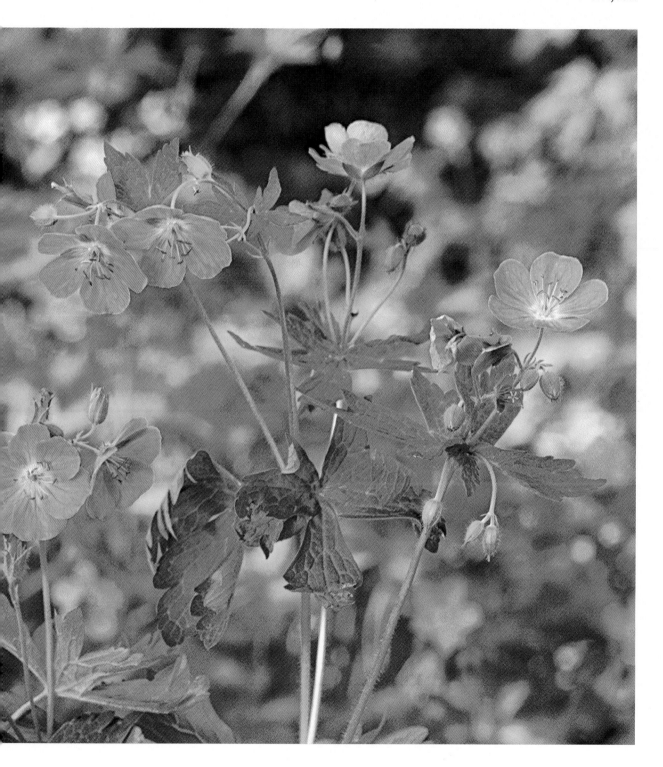

Origins and history

Essential oils have been used since ancient times in a variety of ways—in religious rituals, as medicines, and as cosmetics and perfumes. Evidence of the use of essential oils has been found throughout the ancient world, in both the East and the West.

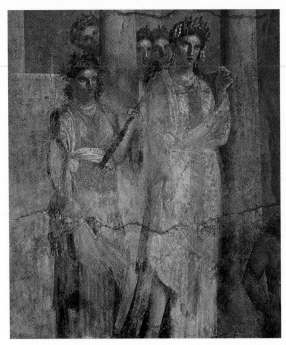

The Romans used essential oils as perfumes, and in massage after bathing.

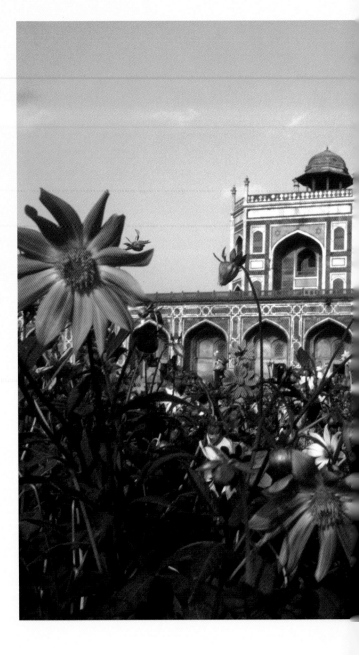

ANCIENT ORIGINS

In the East, plants have been used medicinally in India and China for thousands of years. In the Western world, the ancient Egyptians used fragrant compounds for ritual, therapeutic, and cosmetic purposes. The Greeks built on this knowledge, and the so-called "father of medicine," Hippocrates, referred to a vast amount of medicinal plants in his writings. Greek doctors shared their expertise with the Romans, who also used essential oils as perfumes and in massage after bathing.

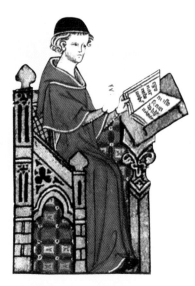

Avicenna (980–1037) was a Persian physician who developed the method of steam distillation.

Medicinal plants have been used in India since ancient times.

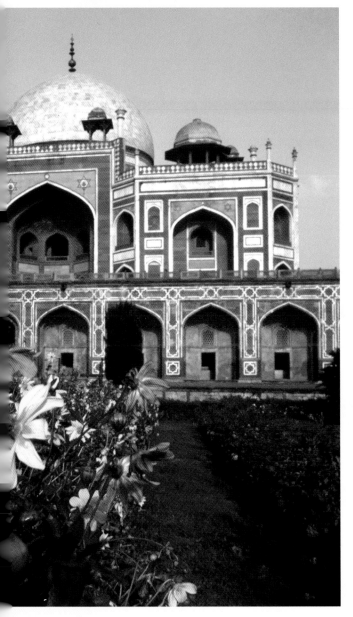

MIDDLE AGES

After the fall of Rome many doctors fled east and their knowledge migrated to the Arabic world. In the 11th century the Persian philosopher and physician Avicenna developed the method of steam distillation. His ideas were brought back to Europe by soldiers returning from the Crusades, and essential oils once again became popular as medicines and perfumes.

MODERN TIMES

During the 19th century the introduction of industrialized production led to a decline in the quality and popularity of essential oils, but they soon returned to favor. When a French chemist, René Gattefossé, burnt his hand in 1910, he applied lavender oil and noticed that the burn healed rapidly with little scarring. This prompted him to study the therapeutic actions of essential oils and he coined the term *aromatherapie* to describe the healing effect of scented oils.

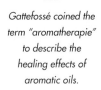

By the 1960s Dr Jean Valnet was using essential oils to treat specific medical and psychiatric disorders, and around the same time Marguerite Maury, a biochemist and beautician, set up the first aromatherapy clinics in Switzerland, France, and Britain. Outside France, the medicinal and therapeutic potential of essential oils has only recently been appreciated, but aromatherapy is now one of the most popular of modern complementary therapies.

Gattefossé coined the term "aromatherapie" to describe the healing effects of aromatic oils.

DRIED CAMOMILE

Camomile oil is extracted from the flowerheads, and can be used to treat various skin complaints.

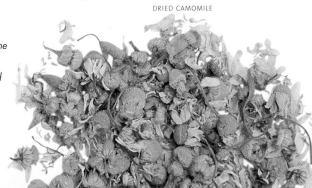

How **oils** enter the **body**

Essential oils are generally absorbed into the body in one of two ways: either through the pores of the skin into the bloodstream during massage, or through nasal cavities during inhalation. Medical aromatherapy, in which oils are taken internally, is not widely practiced outside France.

The speed at which an essential oil is absorbed into the body depends upon the oil being used, air temperature, and the temperature of the oil itself (warmth speeds up absorption). Essential oils are eliminated after several hours, through exhalation and in waste products and perspiration.

INHALATION

Inhaling an essential oil is the quickest way of drawing it into the system. When an aromatic essence is inhaled, it warms and evaporates and gives off its aroma. The vapor dissolves in mucous produced by the mucous membranes in the nasal cavities. This vapor diffuses over microscopic hairs called cilia that convert smells into electrical impulses and transmit them to the brain, specifically the limbic system—this is the part of the brain concerned with basic emotions, memories, and instincts. The limbic system then sends chemical messages, which travel via the nervous system, to give instructions to the rest of the body. A small amount of inhaled oil passes into the lungs and takes part in the gaseous exchange between the air sacs (alveoli) of the lungs and the capillaries of the bloodstream and enters the circulatory system.

THROUGH THE SKIN

Minute essential oil molecules can easily penetrate the skin's layers. Once in the dermis (the layer of skin that gives it its elasticity), they can enter the blood vessels and be transported around the body via the circulatory system.

INTERNAL ADMINISTRATION

When taken internally, essential oils are absorbed through the digestive tract directly into the bloodstream and straight to the liver. This means that the entire dose enters the system at once. There is a risk of irritation and damage to the lining of the intestines, and the oil itself may be toxic. For this reason, essential oils should be administered orally only if prescribed by a qualified and experienced practitioner.

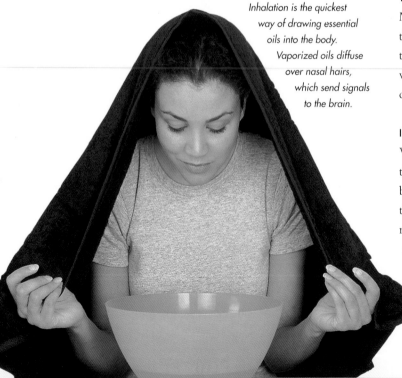

Inhalation is the quickest way of drawing essential oils into the body. Vaporized oils diffuse over nasal hairs, which send signals to the brain.

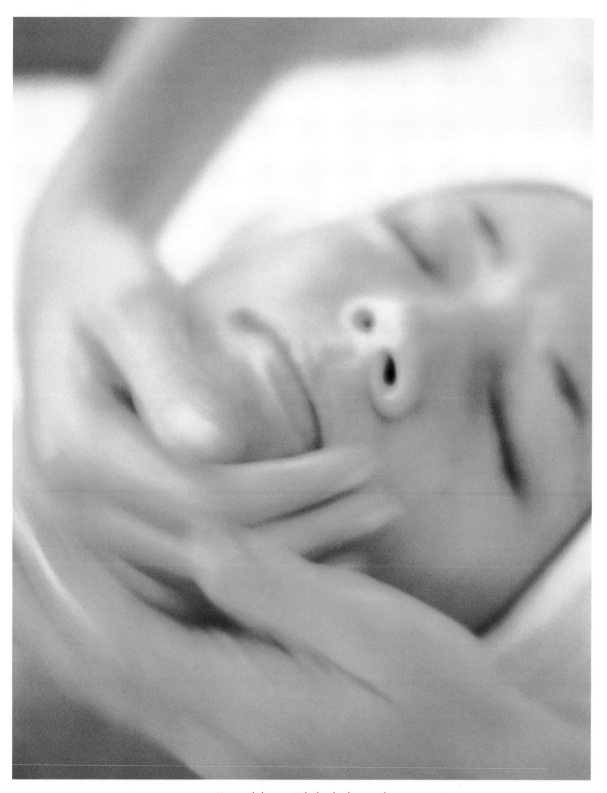

*Massage helps essential oil molecules enter the
pores of the skin, and from there they are
absorbed into the body's bloodstream.*

Benefits of essential oils

Essential oils can relax the mind and the body. They can relieve pain, and restore body systems to a state of equilibrium in which healing can take place. In addition, one of the best things about using essential oils is that they are pleasurable as well as therapeutic, which is another way they can enhance our feelings of well-being.

OILS IN ACTION

The chemical components of essential oils react with body chemistry in a way similar to conventional drugs but with fewer side-effects. Certain essential oils have known physiological effects on the body—for example, rose oil has an effect on many of the hormones involved in reproduction, and others such as lavender are known as adaptogens because they do whatever is required of them at the time. The psychological benefits of essential oils are felt when the aromatic molecules reach the limbic system, the part of the brain that controls emotions and hormones.

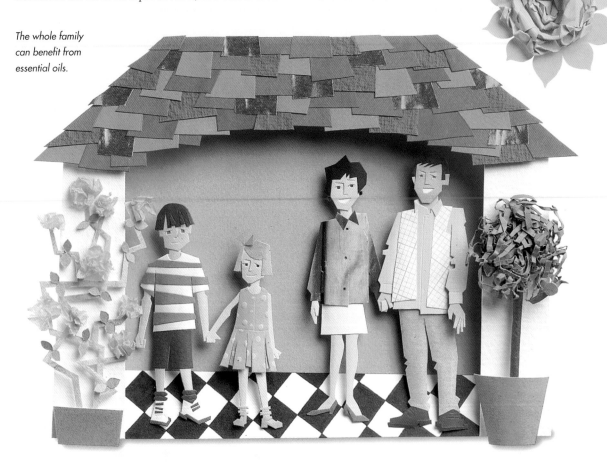

The whole family can benefit from essential oils.

THE ENDOCRINE SYSTEM

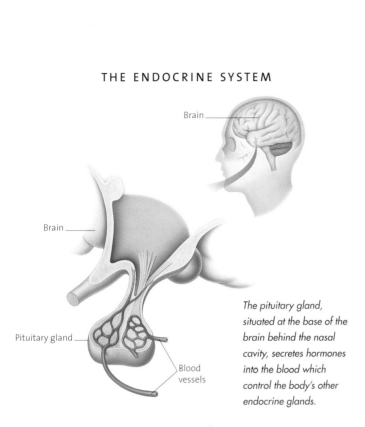

Brain

Brain

Pituitary gland

Blood vessels

The pituitary gland, situated at the base of the brain behind the nasal cavity, secretes hormones into the blood which control the body's other endocrine glands.

HORMONAL ACTION

The aromas released by essential oils influence the endocrine system—a group of glands that produce hormones which regulate metabolism, reproduction, growth, our stress response, and the levels of nutrients in the bloodstream. Some essential oils contain plant hormones that act in a similar manner to our own hormones, reinforcing their effect. Fennel, for example, contains the plant hormone estrogen, which stimulates breast milk production.

FIGHTING INFECTION

Essential oils stimulate the immune system and help the body fight infection by improving the ability of white blood cells to dispose of invading bacteria.

PURIFYING THE BLOOD

Many essential oils purify the blood by stimulating the processes of elimination, which means that toxins that might otherwise lead to a variety of diseases are removed from the system. This is of great benefit for chronic diseases, such as arthritis, and skin problems.

With the aid of a qualified professional, some essential oils can be used in pregnancy to promote well-being.

Preparing essential oils

GERANIUM

A single oil has a unique chemical make-up comprising hundreds of different constituents. Some of these components work synergistically together, meaning that the combination is more effective than an isolated constituent.

METHODS OF EXTRACTION

An essential oil is usually produced by one of the following methods:

Steam distillation The parts of the plant to be used are placed in a container and boiling water or steam is added to break down the plant's cell walls and release the oils. The released essence combines with the steam and is forced into an outlet pipe, which carries away the vapors produced through a condenser system into another vessel. The oil floats on top and is drawn off. The remaining liquid is sometimes recovered for use as a flower water.

Expression Methods of expression vary from crushing the entire fruit to machine abrasion of the outer rind to squeeze out the oils.

Solvent extraction Solvents penetrate the plant tissue and dissolve out the essential oil. An absolute is created by adding alcohol, but the solvent can never be completely removed from the oil extracted.

Carbon dioxide extraction This uses carbon dioxide to explode the plant's molecules and release the oil, but the equipment required is expensive.

STEAM DISTILLATION

In steam distillation, oil is drawn off a plant's vaporized essence after it has been heated.

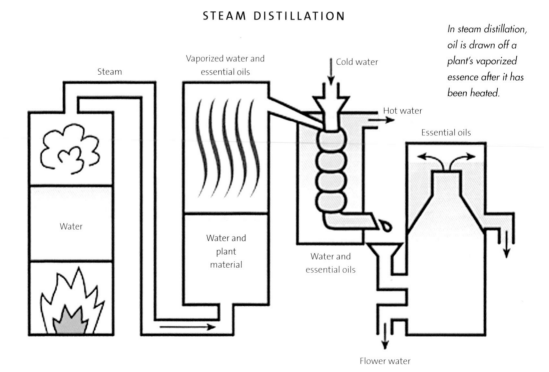

Steam

Vaporized water and essential oils

Cold water

Hot water

Essential oils

Water

Water and plant material

Water and essential oils

Flower water

CHEMICAL COMPONENTS

Most essential oil components are either hydrocarbons (terpenes) or oxygenated compounds. A basic knowledge of the oils' properties and composition will help you to understand how they work.

Terpenes are hydrogen and carbon molecules that combine rapidly with oxygen from the air. This triggers a chain reaction known as oxidation which alters the odor and therapeutic properties of the essential oil. Oils rich in terpenes, such as lemon oil, deteriorate quickly.

Oxygenated compounds belong to different chemical families, including phenols and aldehydes (which often irritate the skin), alcohols, esters, lactones, and ketones. They are less prone to oxidation than terpenes and tend to have a strong smell. Good examples are thyme and rosemary.

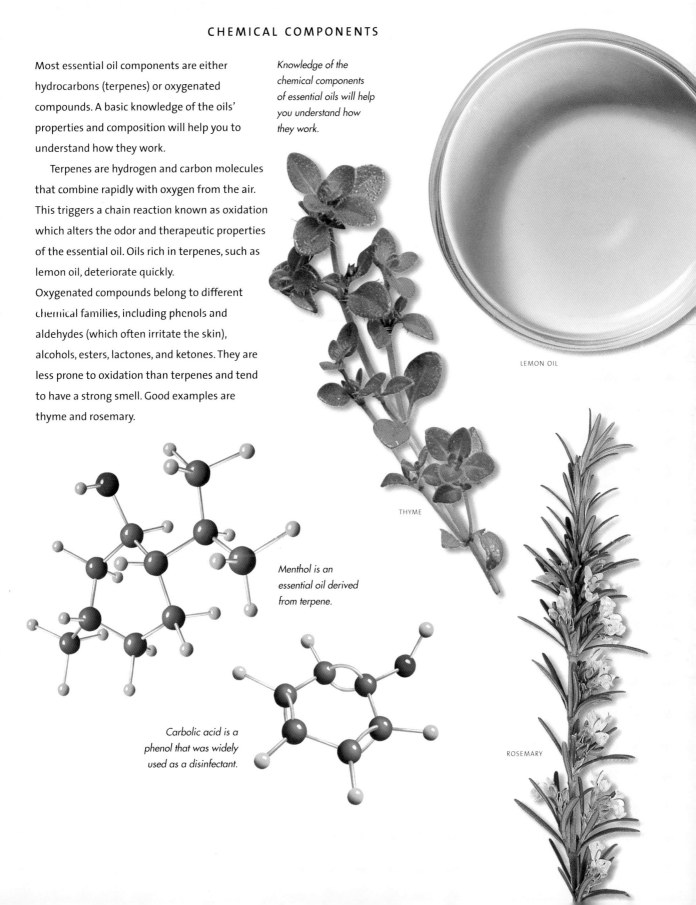

Knowledge of the chemical components of essential oils will help you understand how they work.

LEMON OIL

THYME

Menthol is an essential oil derived from terpene.

Carbolic acid is a phenol that was widely used as a disinfectant.

ROSEMARY

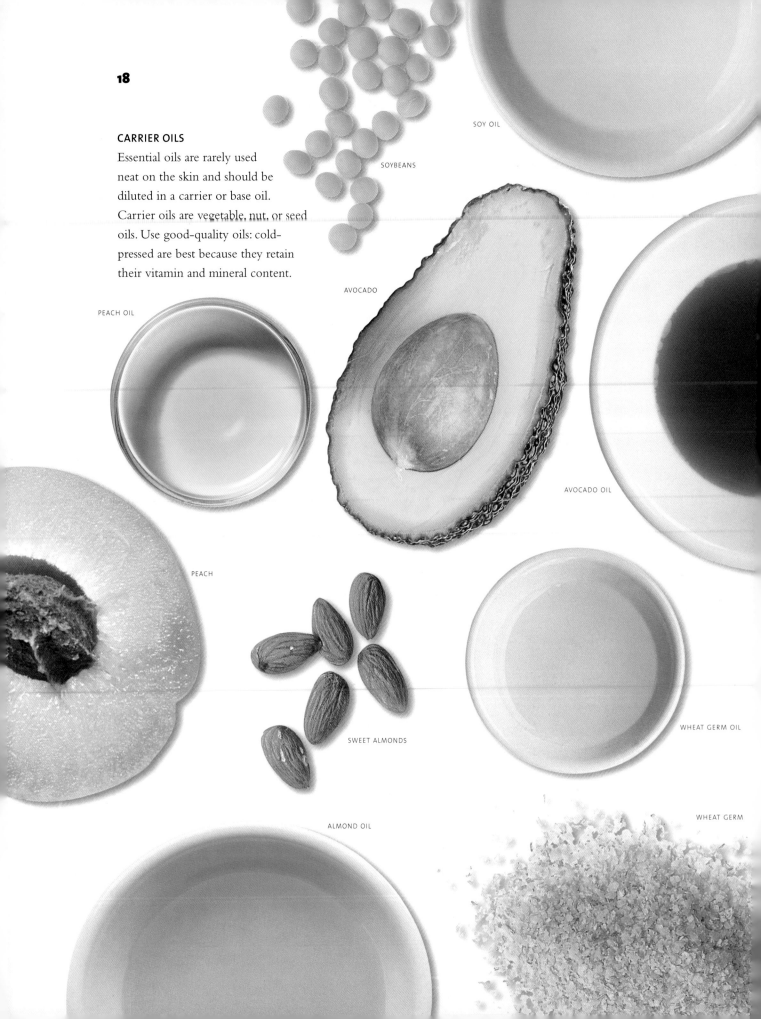

SOY OIL

SOYBEANS

CARRIER OILS

Essential oils are rarely used
neat on the skin and should be
diluted in a carrier or base oil.
Carrier oils are vegetable, nut, or seed
oils. Use good-quality oils: cold-
pressed are best because they retain
their vitamin and mineral content.

AVOCADO

PEACH OIL

AVOCADO OIL

PEACH

SWEET ALMONDS

WHEAT GERM OIL

ALMOND OIL

WHEAT GERM

BLENDING

Oils can be blended to create a different fragrance, or to change the molecular structure of the oils so that they work more effectively. With practice, you will gain the confidence and ability to create pleasing blends.

• Use only a tiny amount of essential oil in proportion to base oil. If you don't like the smell, throw it away and start again.

• The best blends are usually a combination of base notes (deep, rich smells, such as sandalwood), middle notes (floral smells, such as rose), and top notes (light and refreshing, such as citrus).

• Blend six drops of essential oil to 1 tablespoon/15–20 ml of base oil to make a sufficient quantity for a full body massage.

• Add the essential oils to the base oil one at a time.

• Don't use too many essential oils in one blend—generally, three or four is sufficient.

• Make a note of your blends so you can learn from experience.

• Shake well and rub a little on the back of your hand to test. Adjust the proportions as required.

• Store in a dark glass bottle, labeled and dated.

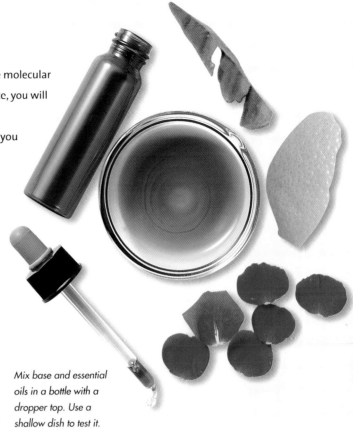

Mix base and essential oils in a bottle with a dropper top. Use a shallow dish to test it.

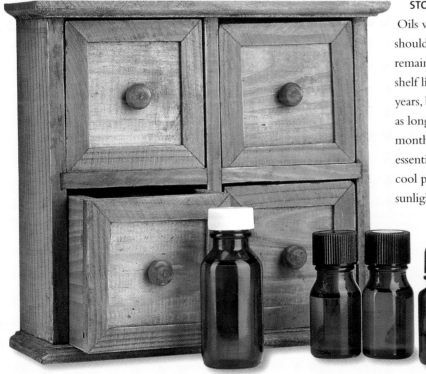

STORING OILS

Oils vary a lot in price and quality, and should be stored carefully to ensure they remain in good condition. The average shelf life of an essential oil is about two years, but when blended it will last only as long as the carrier oil (roughly six months). Light, heat, and oxygen cause essential oils to deteriorate. Store in a cool place, in dark bottles to protect from sunlight. Use small bottles—every time a bottle is opened, oxygen enters and starts to oxidize the oil.

Blended oils should be stored in small, dark bottles in a cool place, to help prevent oxidation.

Precautions

Certain essential oils, such as thyme, clary sage, and rosemary, should be avoided during pregnancy.

Essential oils are safe, enjoyable, and therapeutic when diluted and used properly. However, exercise caution. Do not take internally unless supervised by an experienced and qualified practitioner. Never apply undiluted oils directly to the skin, unless you are certain they are completely non-toxic. Avoid rosemary and Scotch pine oil if you have high blood pressure.

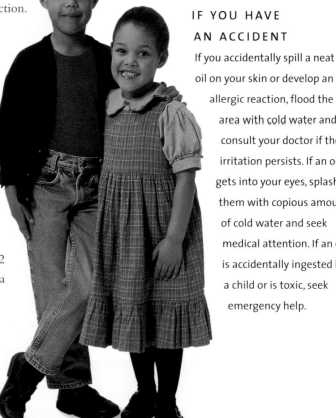

For sensitive skin, use an adhesive bandage to do a patch test for 24 hours.

If you have sensitive skin, do a patch test first. Apply the diluted oil to a small patch of skin on your wrist or elbow. Cover with an adhesive bandage and leave for 24 hours to see if an irritation develops. Do not use if there is an adverse reaction.

BABIES AND CHILDREN

Treat essential oils as you would medicines and keep them in a cupboard well out of children's reach. Mandarin, myrtle, lavender, and Roman camomile can be used in a vaporizer for the benefit of babies, but should not be used diluted on the skin until the child is at least a year old. Children are very sensitive to the properties of essential oils and the dosage has to be much smaller: add one drop to 2 teaspoons/10 ml of sweet almond oil for a massage and carry out a patch test first.

Children and babies can benefit from essential oils, but the concentration must be much smaller.

PREGNANCY

Oils such as mandarin and rose are perfectly safe to use externally during pregnancy, but are generally used in a low dilution (five drops of essential oil per 4 teaspoons/20 ml of carrier oil). Many oils regulate the menstrual cycle and must be avoided in pregnancy—thyme, clary sage, and rosemary in particular. If in any doubt, do not use.

IF YOU HAVE AN ACCIDENT

If you accidentally spill a neat oil on your skin or develop an allergic reaction, flood the area with cold water and consult your doctor if the irritation persists. If an oil gets into your eyes, splash them with copious amounts of cold water and seek medical attention. If an oil is accidentally ingested by a child or is toxic, seek emergency help.

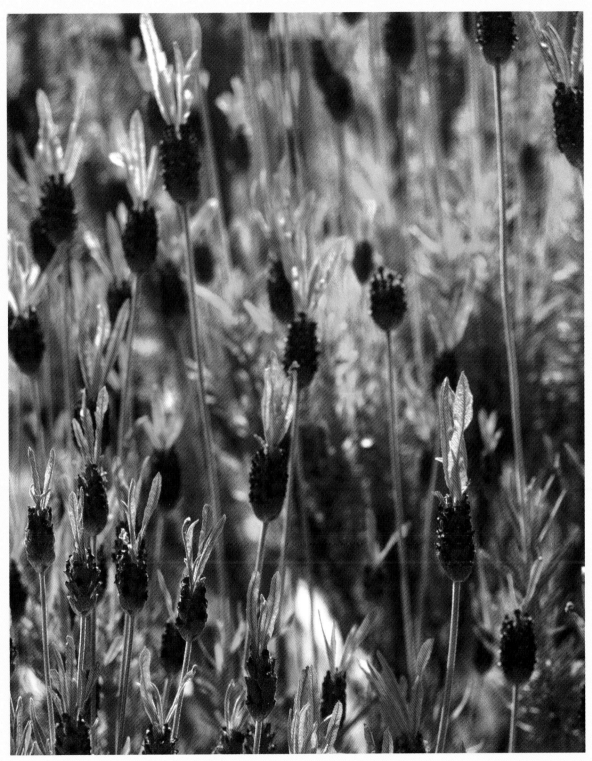

*Lavender oil can be used to help treat
allergies, eczema, dermatitis, and wounds,
but it should not be used on the skin of
children under a year old.*

How to use essential oils

There are many effective ways of using essential oils. The most popular and relaxing way is to apply diluted oils in a body massage, but other methods are just as suitable.

BATHS

Adding oils to the bath is a pleasurable way of using them. Add to the water once the bath has been run, as the heat causes them to evaporate. The warm water promotes relaxation and helps the oils to penetrate the skin. Use neat essential oils only if they are completely non-irritant. Lavender and marjoram are good, non-irritant oils. Otherwise, dilute in a base oil.

BURNERS AND VAPORIZERS

These include saucers, lightbulb rings, and radiator diffusers, but the most common are ceramic pots warmed by a small candle. Add water and a few drops of oil to the vaporizer. Remember never to leave a naked flame unattended and to use an electric vaporizer during the night.

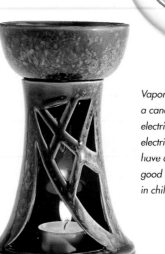

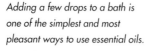

Vaporizers can be heated by a candle flame (left) or by electricity (above). Since electric vaporizers do not have a naked flame, they are good for night use, especially in children's bedrooms.

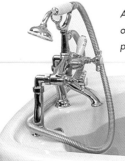

Adding a few drops to a bath is one of the simplest and most pleasant ways to use essential oils.

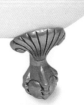

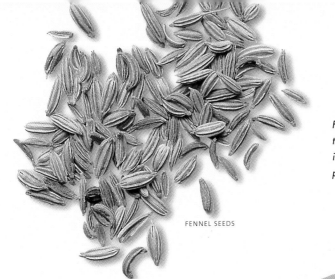

Fennel oil is extracted from the crushed seeds. Lemon oil is extracted from the outer part of the fresh peel.

FENNEL SEEDS

LEMON

COMPRESSES

A hot compress is an effective way of treating complaints such as skin infections (including boils) and muscle pain. Pour hot water into a bowl and add four or five drops of the essential oil. Soak a clean cloth in the water and squeeze out the excess water. Apply immediately to the affected area and keep warm by wrapping a towel around it. Keep the compress in place for about an hour.

A cold compress is good for headaches, swellings, and sprains. Pour cold water into a bowl and add some ice cubes. Add some drops of essential oil, then dip your cloth into it and place over the affected part.

COOKING

Essential oils, such as lemon and fennel, have been used as flavorings for thousands of years. Add one or two drops to the liquid when cooking.

GARGLES AND MOUTHWASHES

These are beneficial for treating sore throats, infections, and mouth ulcers. Dilute two or three drops of essential oil in strong alcohol (vodka or brandy). Add to a small glass of warm water and use as a gargle or swish around the mouth. Do not swallow.

Essential oils can be used to enhance the flavor of salad dressings and sauces.

Tea tree oil added to a glass of warm water and gargled daily helps treat mouth ulcers.

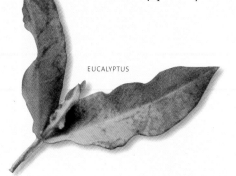

EUCALYPTUS

Inhalations of eucalyptus oil help asthma, coughs, and throat infections.

INHALATIONS

Inhalations are very effective for coughs, colds, and sore throats, but they are not suitable for people with breathing difficulties or asthma, and should not be used for treating children. Add three or four drops of oil (two or three of peppermint or eucalyptus) to a bowl of steaming water. Lean over the bowl, then place a large towel over your head and breathe deeply for a few minutes.

Alternatively, place four or five drops of oil on a tissue, then hold it to your nose and inhale. Never inhale directly from the bottle, unless the oil is specifically described as safe to use in this way, probably for first aid.

EUCALYPTUS

Add a few drops of oil to a bowl of steaming water, then cover your head with a towel and breathe deeply for a few minutes, keeping your eyes closed.

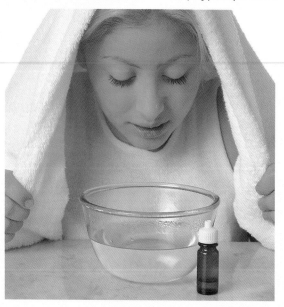

MASSAGE

With an aromatherapy massage, you get the benefit of the massage as well as the benefits of the essential oils. The rubbing action ensures the oils are well absorbed into the skin. Massage is the method preferred by aromatherapists. DO NOT USE UNDILUTED OILS DIRECTLY ON SKIN.

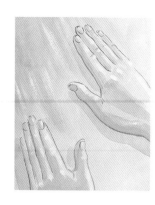

1 Long, sweeping strokes known as effleurage help to spread the oils across the skin. They are ideal for use at the beginning of a massage and in between deeper strokes.

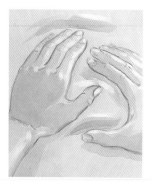

2 Lifting areas of skin and rolling them in the palm is known as kneading. This stimulates the circulation, relieves muscle tension, and improves skin tone.

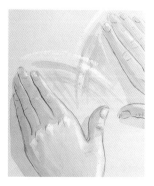

3 Working the thumbs in small, circling movements with deep pressure, known as petrissage, eases knotted muscles and helps to relieve tension in the body.

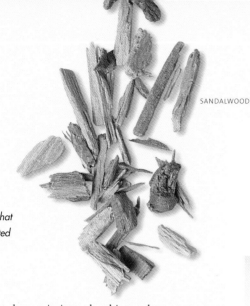

SANDALWOOD

Sandalwood has a musky, sweet scent that can be worn undiluted on the skin.

PERFUMES

Essential oils that do not irritate the skin, such as lavender, jasmine, sandalwood, and rose, may be worn undiluted as perfumes—dab a drop on your pulse points. They are subtle and long-lasting, and do not have a cloying, alcoholic base.

SPRAYS

To make a room spray, half-fill a plant spray with water, then add 10 drops of essential oil. Shake well, then spray liberally, making sure it does not come into contact with your skin. Sprays can be used to disinfect and fumigate a sickroom, add fragrance, or repel insects. Adding calming oil can make a room more relaxing.

TOILETRIES

You can create a range of lotions and potions at home using your favorite essential oils.

HOW TO MAKE SCENTED SOAP

You will need:

8 fl oz/225 ml each of carrier oil, water, and unscented vegetable soap flakes; three essential oils of your choice.

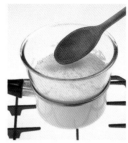

1 Place all the ingredients in a heatproof bowl over a pan of hot water and leave until the soap flakes have dissolved.

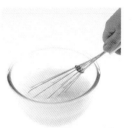

2 Remove the bowl from the heat and whisk to make sure the ingredients are well-blended.

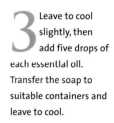

3 Leave to cool slightly, then add five drops of each essential oil. Transfer the soap to suitable containers and leave to cool.

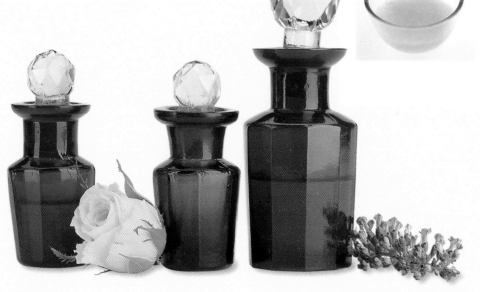

You can make a selection of perfumes using your favorite essential oils, and those perfumes will be highly individual.

Directory of oils

The following pages provide a fully illustrated guide to 46 of the most common and safe essential oils. The oils are listed alphabetically by their botanical names. Each profile gives a list of the main characteristics and properties of the oil, along with details of the ways in which it may be used. There are also recommendations for good blending.

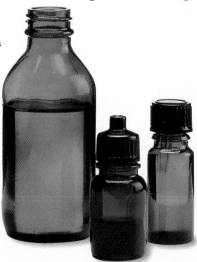

Use the following pages to select the oils you want to blend.

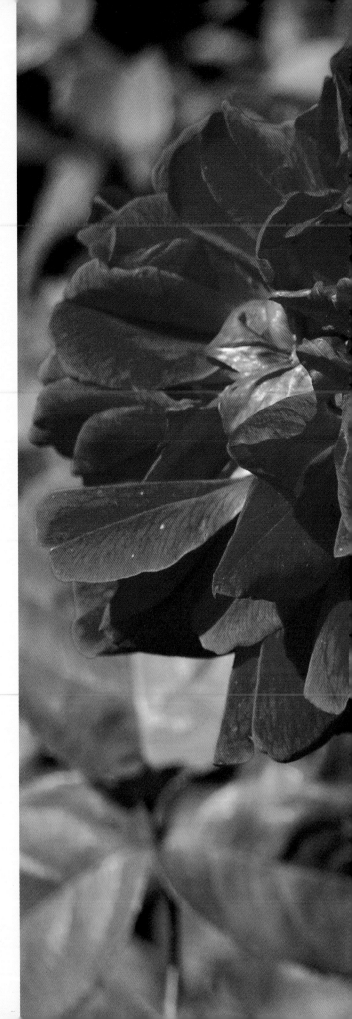

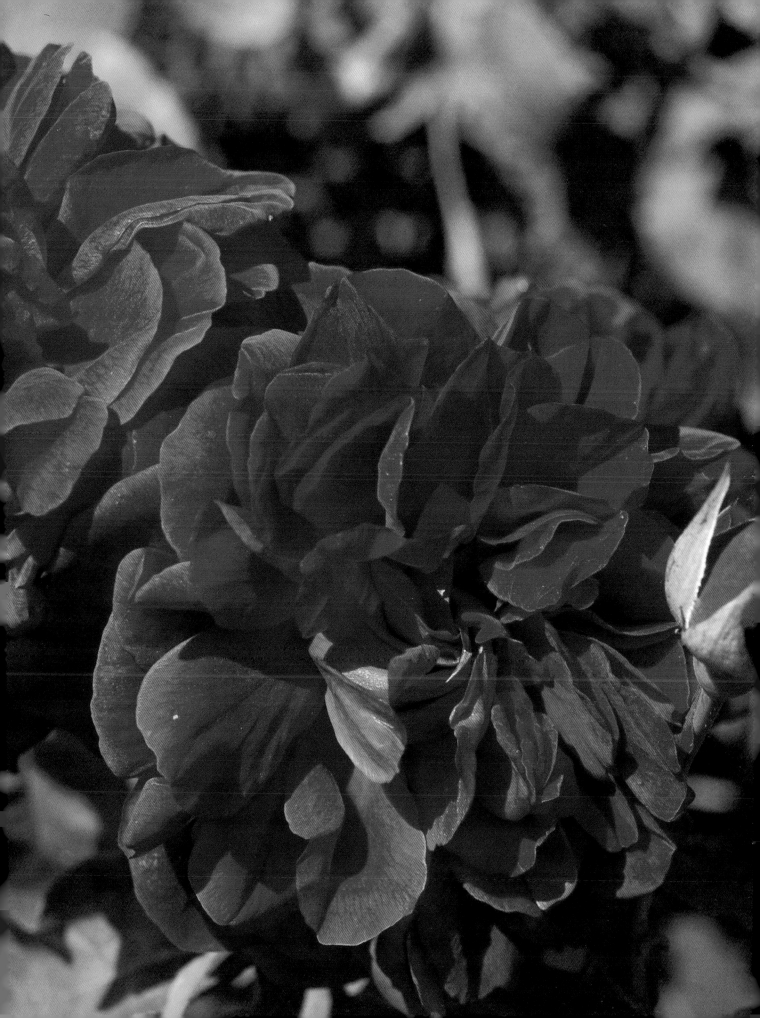

Yarrow Achillea millefolium

Yarrow can be used to treat dry skin, eczema, or rashes.

Associated with divination, yarrow was used by the Druids to predict the weather, and in China the stalks are still used when consulting the *I Ching* (*Book of Changes*). The essential oil is distilled from the dried flower heads and has a sweet, spicy scent.

KEY PROPERTIES AND CHARACTERISTICS

Anti-inflammatory, revitalizing, febrifugal, balancing, relieves indigestion, diuretic.

BLENDS

Blends well with angelica, cedarwood, rosemary, vetiver, and lemon oils.

In ancient China, yarrow stalks were used alongside the Book of Changes to try and predict the future.

USES

Yarrow essential oil contains azulene, an anti-inflammatory, and alleviates muscle pain and headaches. It is effective for treating high blood pressure and irregular or heavy periods. Yarrow helps to settle a nervous stomach and can alleviate diarrhea and flatulence. It promotes the skin's natural healing process, being beneficial for wounds, ulcers, and dry skin. Yarrow increases perspiration and is beneficial for feverish illnesses, especially colds and influenza. It also elevates mood and promotes restful sleep.

CAUTION
May increase the skin's sensitivity to sunlight, and cause allergic rashes or headaches.

Yarrow has finely dissected leaves with many dense, pinkish-white flowerheads.

Angelica Angelica archangelica

This bitter-sweet, large, hairy aromatic plant, often used to flavor gin, was valued as a medieval panacea. The root and seeds are distilled to produce the essential oil, which has an earthy, sweet, woody scent.

Angelica is a large, hairy plant with broad, bright green leaves and stems.

KEY PROPERTIES AND CHARACTERISTICS

Revitalizing, detoxifying, diuretic, expectorant, antispasmodic, anti-inflammatory, stimulant.

ANGELICA ROOT

BLENDS

Blends well with clary sage, camomile, vetiver, and citrus oils.

USES

Used to strengthen the immune system and speed up the healing of cuts and bruises. Angelica's detoxifying and diuretic properties make it effective for treating cellulite, arthritis, and fluid retention. It relieves digestive disorders caused by stress and is beneficial for indigestion, colic, nausea, and flatulence. Angelica brings rapid pain relief and can alleviate cases of headache, migraine, and toothache. It is also beneficial in treating colds, bronchitis, and respiratory infections.

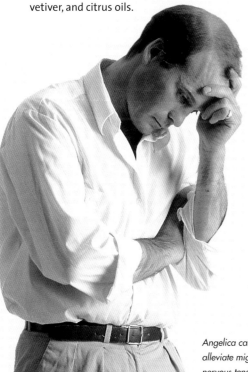

Angelica can help alleviate migraine, nervous tension, and stress-related disorders.

CAUTION
Do not use in pregnancy or if you are diabetic. Angelica may increase the skin's sensitivity to sunlight.

Rosewood Aniba rosaeodora

Cultivation of the rosewood is contributing to the destruction of the South American rainforests, so use sparingly and try to ensure your supply comes from a sustainable source. The essential oil, which has a sweet, floral, woody scent, is extracted from wood chippings.

Rosewood oil is extracted by steam distillation of the tree's wood chippings.

KEY PROPERTIES AND CHARACTERISTICS

Antidepressant, anti-inflammatory, aphrodisiac, deodorizing, deeply relaxing without being sedative, immune system stimulant, tonic.

BLENDS

Blends well with bergamot, cedarwood, clove, rose, frankincense, lemon, mandarin, and sandalwood.

Rosewood oil is good for skin care because it stimulates tissue regeneration. It can help treat acne, dermatitis, scars, and wrinkles.

USES

This oil is safe to use for children's ailments. It has a mild, tonifying effect on the nervous system and is both calming and uplifting. Rosewood boosts the immune system and deals effectively with infections and viruses. The oil relieves stress and tension headaches, and is suitable for treating disorders caused by stress. It may help to restore libido if sexual dysfunction is caused by emotional problems. Rosewood is also a useful skincare product because it stimulates cell growth and tissue regeneration, helping to diminish wrinkles and scars.

Frankincense Boswellia carteri

Frankincense has been used for cosmetic and medicinal purposes, and as an incense, for thousands of years. The tree grows wild in North Africa, and the oil, extracted from gum resin, has a long-lasting, sweet, spicy aroma.

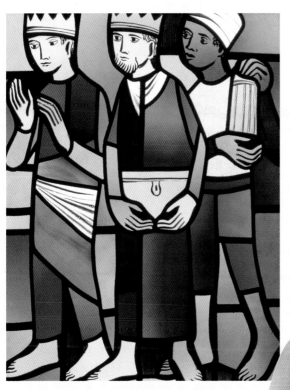

Frankincense has been used in medicines and as an incense since ancient times. In the Bible, one of the three wise men brought Jesus a gift of frankincense, as depicted here.

USES

The main effect of frankincense is on the nervous system, and it is calming and uplifting. Frankincense effectively relieves anxiety and nervous tension, emotional upsets, and stress-related digestive disorders. It has a soothing effect on the mucous membranes and is particularly effective in clearing the nasal passages. Its tonifying and rejuvenating properties make frankincense beneficial for improving skin tone and treating aging skin. Frankincense can ease period pains and urinary tract infections such as cystitis. Its antiseptic and astringent properties make it useful for healing wounds.

BLENDS

Blends well with rose, lavender, geranium, citrus oils, sandalwood, pine, spice oils, and vetiver.

Frankincense is calming and uplifting. It can help to relieve anxiety, nervous tension, emotional upsets, and stress-related conditions.

KEY PROPERTIES AND CHARACTERISTICS

Anti-inflammatory, antiseptic, astringent, diuretic, expectorant, sedative, tonic, uplifting, uterine tonic.

DRIED YLANG YLANG

Ylang ylang Cananga odorata

Ylang ylang oil is produced from the freshly picked flowers of a semi-wild, tropical evergreen tree, sometimes known as the perfume tree. It is found mainly in Indonesia and the Philippines. One tree produces about 265 lb/120 kg flowers, which yield 12 oz/350 g of essential oil. The oil has a very powerful, sweet, exotic scent with a balsamic undertone.

KEY PROPERTIES AND CHARACTERISTICS

Antidepressant, antiseptic, aphrodisiac, euphoric, sedative, soothing, stimulant, tonic.

USES

This calming, soothing oil is very effective for treating problems caused by anxiety, stress-related disorders, tension, and depression. Ylang ylang has a well-established reputation as an aphrodisiac. It is useful for treating high blood pressure, palpitations, circulatory disorders, panic attacks, and shock. It is often sniffed from the bottle like smelling salts for first aid. It can also be used in general skin care.

CAUTION

Do not use if skin is inflamed. Excessive use may cause headaches or nausea.

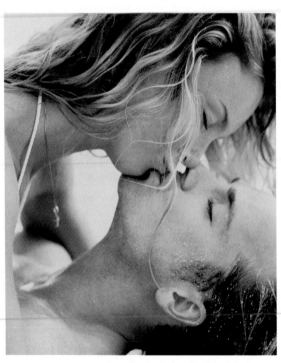

Ylang ylang is well known for its aphrodisiac effect. It has a heady, sensual scent and can induce euphoria.

Leaves from a ylang ylang tree, which can grow up to 68 ft/20 m high.

BLENDS

The oil becomes more powerful when mixed with others. Bergamot, jasmine, lemon, lavender, rose, rosewood, and sandalwood are good for blending.

CEDARWOOD
PINE

Atlas cedarwood

Cedrus atlantica

The pine cones of the Atlas cedar, like the rest of the wood, have a rich, sweet smell.

Atlas cedarwood was one of the earliest oils to be extracted and was used by the ancient Egyptians for embalming their dead. The oil is distilled from the wood and sawdust, and has a sweet, rich smell that becomes more woody as it dries out.

The leaves of Atlas cedars are blue-green pine needles. The trees grow up to 120 ft /35 m tall.

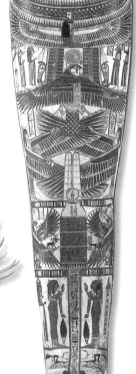

The ancient Egyptians used cedarwood oil to embalm their dead.

USES

Oily hair and skin, acne, dandruff, and fungal infections such as athlete's foot respond well to cedarwood. It has a reputation for stimulating hair growth and may alleviate hair loss. Coughs and bronchial congestion are relieved by its expectorant properties. Chronic conditions such as arthritis benefit from cedarwood's regenerative properties. Cedarwood helps to relieve cystitis, and has a diuretic action that reduces cellulite and water retention. It has a calming, soothing effect, and helps to relieve nervous tension.

CAUTION

Do not use during pregnancy.

KEY PROPERTIES AND CHARACTERISTICS

Aphrodisiac, uplifting, reviving, warming, comforting, stimulating, tonifying, soothing, diuretic, expectorant, and mildly astringent.

BLENDS

Blends well with bergamot, cypress, frankincense, jasmine, juniper, myrrh, neroli, rosemary, sandalwood, and vetiver.

Roman camomile

Chamaemelum nobile

Camomile can help treat eczema, acne, dermatitis, and inflamed skin conditions.

This daisy-like plant is an ancient healing herb, traditionally used for stress-related and digestive disorders. Camomile tea aids digestion and promotes restful sleep. The oil, which has a sweet, grassy smell with a fruity undertone, is extracted from the flowerheads.

KEY PROPERTIES AND CHARACTERISTICS

Soothing, antidepressant, anti-allergenic, anti-inflammatory, antiseptic, bactericidal, mild sedative.

USES

This gentle oil can be used for treating children's ailments. Camomile calms the nervous system and eases headaches, stress, irritability, and nervousness, and is known to promote sleep. Camomile is suitable for treating stress-related digestive disorders, and has pain-relieving properties. It is particularly effective when treating allergies, and itchy and inflamed skin conditions. Camomile relieves PMS and helps regulate periods. It stimulates white blood cell production and boosts the immune system: good for treating viruses or infections.

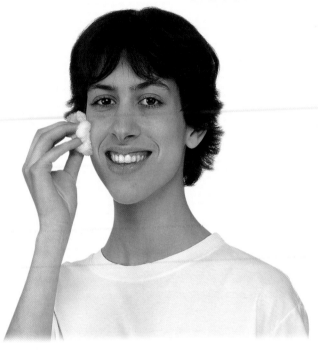

BLENDS

Blends well with clary sage, lavender, lemon, marjoram, and rose.

CAUTION

Do not use in the first trimester of pregnancy.

Camomile oil is extracted from the flowerheads by steam distillation.

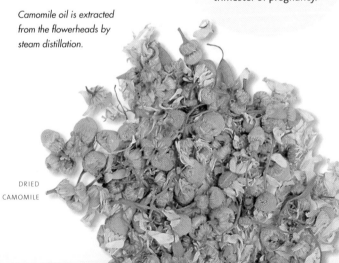

DRIED CAMOMILE

Cinnamon leaf

Cinnamomum zeylanicum

Oil extracted from the leaves is non-toxic, but it could be a skin irritant.

Cinnamon is one of the oldest known and most commercially important spices, with recorded use in China in 2700 BCE. The essential oil used in aromatherapy is distilled from the leaves and young twigs and has a warm, spicy odor.

Cinnamon oil can be distilled from the twigs or leaves of the tropical tree.

DRIED CINNAMON

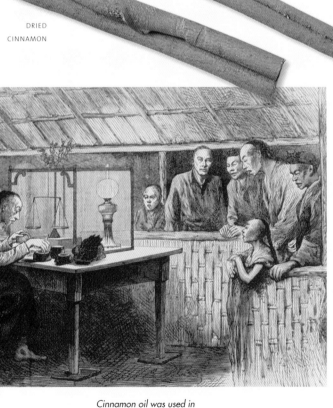

Cinnamon oil was used in ancient Chinese medicine over 4,000 years ago.

USES

Cinnamon strengthens and tonifies the circulatory, respiratory, and digestive systems. Its powerful antiseptic properties make it good for treating colds and flu. It is a useful parasiticide for treating head lice and scabies. Cinnamon stimulates a sluggish digestion and relieves digestive spasms and flatulence. It can be used to treat rheumatism, and may elevate mood and improve concentration.

CAUTION

Do not confuse with cinnamon bark oil, which is an extreme irritant and should not be used as an essential oil. Do not use in concentrations of more than 0.5 per cent, carry out a patch test before using, and never use on the face.

KEY PROPERTIES AND CHARACTERISTICS

Warming, stimulating, uplifting, tonifying, aphrodisiac, antispasmodic, and antiseptic.

BLENDS

Blends well with eucalyptus, clove, frankincense, and citrus oils.

Lime Citrus aurantiifolia

Limes are a traditional remedy for indigestion and were used by sailors in the 18th century to prevent scurvy. The essential oil is expressed from the peel or distilled from the whole fruit, and it has a light, sweet, rich scent.

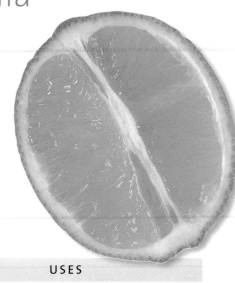

Lime oil can be distilled from the whole, ripe fruit when it is crushed.

KEY PROPERTIES AND CHARACTERISTICS

Antioxidant, antiseptic, aromatic, astringent, cooling, deodorizing, disinfectant, febrifugal, tonic, and apéritif.

BLENDS

Lime blends well with lavender, rosemary, other citrus oils, clary sage, and bergamot.

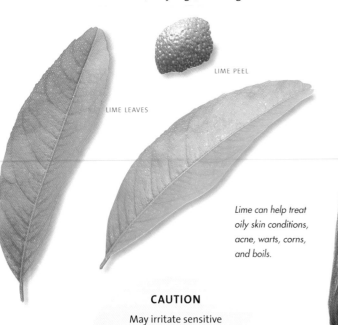

LIME PEEL

LIME LEAVES

Lime can help treat oily skin conditions, acne, warts, corns, and boils.

CAUTION

May irritate sensitive skin and increase the skin's sensitivity to sunlight.

USES

Limes have similar properties to lemons and the two are often used interchangeably. Lime acts as an immune system tonic and is refreshing and stimulating, good for tiredness, apathy, and depression. It acts as a digestive stimulant. Its antiseptic, bactericidal, and febrifugal properties make it beneficial in cooling fever and fighting respiratory infections. It can help relieve the pain of rheumatism and arthritis. Lime's astringent properties are helpful for oily skin and conditions such as boils and acne.

Neroli Citrus aurantium

Neroli flowers (orange blossom) are traditionally included in bridal bouquets to calm nervous brides. The oil is produced from the flowers of the bitter or Seville orange tree, and is a classic perfume and eau de Cologne ingredient. Neroli oil has a powerful, floral, sweet aroma, which is also light and refreshing.

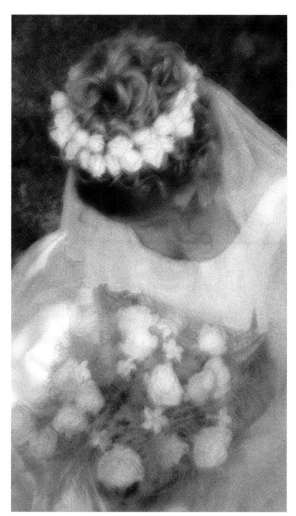

The white blossoms of the neroli tree are still used in bridal bouquets today. Its calming quality soothes nervous brides.

USES

The main action of neroli is on the nervous system, and it is a very effective antidepressant. It promotes relaxation and sleep, and helps to clear the mind and lift the spirits. Neroli oil has diuretic effects and regulates blood pressure. It also reduces inflammation and controls bacterial and fungal infections. Neroli eases digestive cramps and stress-related diarrhea. Dry, aging skin, wrinkles, and broken blood vessels benefit from neroli's rejuvenating properties, and it might help to prevent stretch marks during pregnancy.

KEY PROPERTIES AND CHARACTERISTICS

Bitter, aromatic, expectorant, antidepressant, aphrodisiac, calming, antispasmodic, rejuvenating.

BLENDS

Blends well with bergamot, clary sage, frankincense, jasmine, lavender, other citrus oils, rose, rosemary, and ylang ylang.

Neroli leaves also produce petitgrain oil, which has similar qualities to neroli oil.

ORANGE PEEL

Orange Citrus aurantium

Orange oil has a long history of use in Traditional Chinese Medicine and is a popular ingredient in the food and drink industry. The oil is expressed from the peel and has a sweet, fresh, fruity fragrance.

KEY PROPERTIES AND CHARACTERISTICS

Versatile, relaxing, uplifting, detoxifying, laxative, balancing, and astringent.

BLENDS

Blends particularly well with spice oils, other citrus oils, clary sage, geranium, lavender, myrrh, neroli, camomile, and rosemary.

Orange oil is extracted from the peel of the fruit. It has a fresh, citrus scent.

USES

This uplifting, relaxing oil is very beneficial when treating conditions caused by stress and nervous exhaustion, including insomnia. Orange oil has a general detoxifying and cleansing effect; it encourages the elimination of excess fluid and waste products, and is useful for counteracting cellulite. Its tonifying and astringent properties make it appropriate for treating oily, dull, tired skin or hair. It can also help treat acne. The main effect of orange oil is to speed up the digestive system and relieve constipation and flatulence. It can also be used to treat gastric fevers, colds, and flu. Orange oil is non-toxic and safe to use for children's ailments.

Other types of orange oil are extracted from the leaves or the flowers.

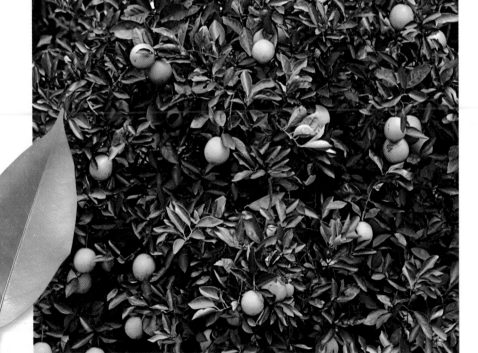

Bergamot
Citrus bergamia

The bergamot orange is similar in appearance to the bitter orange, but with small yellow fruit. The oil, which has a refreshing, sweet, fruity smell, is extracted from the fruit peel. Bergamot oil gives Earl Grey tea its distinctive flavor, and is the main constituent of eau de Cologne.

Bergamot oil is extracted from the peel of the nearly ripe fruit, which look like small oranges.

Bergamot is the distinctive flavoring used in Earl Grey tea. It has a fresh, sweet, fruity scent and balsamic undertones.

USES

Bergamot oil is widely used in a douche to treat genito-urinary infections such as cystitis. Oily skin conditions, eczema, psoriasis, cuts, acne, and boils respond well to bergamot. The oil limits viral activity and can be used to treat cold sores, chickenpox, and shingles.

It is a powerful antidepressant, is helpful during times of stress, and may relieve tension headaches. Its carminative and antispasmodic properties make it beneficial for digestive disorders such as flatulence and indigestion.

KEY PROPERTIES AND CHARACTERISTICS

Cooling, calming, reviving, refreshing, uplifting, tonic, soothing, carminative, antiseptic, and antidepressant.

BLENDS

Blends well with cypress, geranium, melissa, neroli, pine, and rosemary.

CAUTION
Avoid if you have sensitive skin. Bergamot increases the skin's sensitivity to sunlight.

Bergamot oil is commonly used to treat cystitis and thrush. It is also helpful for stress-related conditions.

Lemon Citrus limon

Native to India, the lemon tree is now cultivated all over the world, and has a long history of use in European folk medicine. The oil is extracted from the outer part of the peel and has a fresh, sharp, citrus smell.

Lemon tree leaves are oval-shaped, with stiff thorns growing below.

USES

This refreshing, cleansing, and tonifying oil is one of the most important oils for treating all kinds of infection. Lemon is a tonic for the circulatory system and is effective in treating varicose veins, sluggish circulation, low blood pressure, and fluid retention. It stimulates the production of red and white blood cells, boosting the immune system and alleviating anemia. Lemon oil cleanses and detoxifies the digestive system, and can be used to treat obesity or loss of appetite. Its astringent properties make it appropriate for treating oily skin and hair conditions.

KEY PROPERTIES AND CHARACTERISTICS

Astringent, antiseptic, cleansing, refreshing, tonic, stimulant, bactericidal, and diuretic.

Lemon oil can help treat all kinds of digestive ailments, including loss of appetite or poor appetite.

BLENDS

Other citrus oils, lavender, ylang ylang, geranium, juniper, eucalyptus, sandalwood, and frankincense.

CAUTION

May irritate sensitive skin.
Avoid sunlight after use.

GRAPEFRUIT PEEL

Grapefruit Citrus paradisi

Like other citrus fruits, this large, yellow fruit is high in vitamin C and cleanses the body's systems. The oil is expressed from the rind of the ripe fruit and has a fresh, tangy, citrus smell. Unlike many citrus oils, grapefruit does not increase the skin's sensitivity to sunlight.

KEY PROPERTIES AND CHARACTERISTICS

Cooling, astringent, tonic, detoxifying, refreshing, antiseptic, and cleansing.

Grapefruit oil is extracted from the fresh peel of the ripe fruit.

GRAPEFRUIT LEAF

BLENDS

Blends well with other citrus oils, clove, cypress, ginger, lavender, palmarosa, rosemary, and other spice oils.

USES

Grapefruit is one of the main essential oils used in the treatment of obesity and can help to reduce the appetite and stimulate the metabolic rate. Because of its detoxifying and diuretic properties, it relieves fluid retention and helps combat cellulite. It has a cooling, detoxifying effect, good for treating hangovers. Its astringent properties make it helpful for acne and oily skin conditions and toning the skin. Grapefruit has a beneficial action on the respiratory system, good for treating colds and flu.

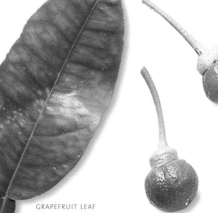

Grapefruit oil's cooling, detoxifying effect makes it good for treating hangovers. It can also be used to treat depression, headaches, nervous exhaustion, or stress.

MANDARIN PEEL

Mandarin Citrus reticulata

Mandarins grow on small evergreen trees with fragrant flowers and glossy leaves. They originate in China, where they were a traditional offering to Chinese rulers (from whom they take their name). Mandarin oil is expressed from the peel of the ripe fruit and has an extremely sweet, fruity, floral smell.

Mandarin oil is extracted from the outer peel of the fleshy fruit.

KEY PROPERTIES AND CHARACTERISTICS

Mildly laxative, soothing, antispasmodic, carminative, diuretic, sedative, detoxifying, and slightly astringent.

CAUTION

May be slightly phototoxic.

BLENDS

Blends well with other citrus oils, spice oils, clary sage, geranium, juniper, lavender, and frankincense.

USES

Mandarin oil is safe to use in pregnancy. It can also be used to treat children's problems such as hiccups, colic, indigestion, or hyperactivity. The main action of mandarin is on the digestive system, and it speeds up digestion and relieves constipation, indigestion, and intestinal spasms. It has a mildly laxative effect. Its sedative properties relieve nervous tension, restlessness, and insomnia. The oil is suitable for treating oily skin conditions, and it can help prevent stretch marks if massaged into the abdominal region during pregnancy.

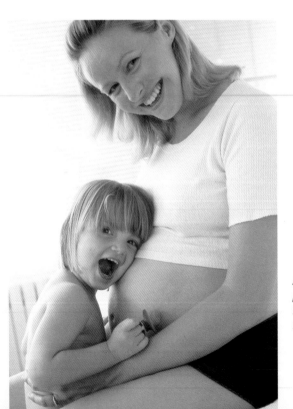

Mandarin oil is safe to use in pregnancy, and can help treat hiccups, colic, indigestion, or hyperactivity in children.

Myrrh Commiphora myrrha

MYRRH

Myrrh has been used since ancient times in embalming, medicine, and as an incense. In the Bible, it was one of the gifts brought by the three wise men to Jesus. The essential oil is extracted from resin in the bark of the tree trunk.

Myrrh is distilled from resin taken from the bark. It has a balsamic, medicinal smell.

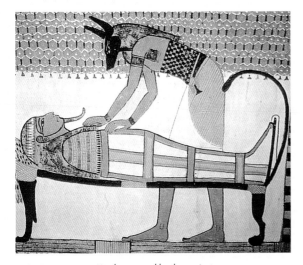

Myrrh was used by the ancient Egyptians for embalming their dead.

CAUTION

Do not use in pregnancy.

USES

Myrrh is an expectorant and tonic for the respiratory system, excellent for treating coughs, colds, and bronchitis. It soothes the digestive system and is appropriate for treating poor digestion and flatulence. Mouth ulcers, sore throats, bad breath, bleeding gums, and wounds benefit from its antiseptic and healing properties. The oil acts as a uterine tonic, alleviating period problems. Myrrh has powerful preservative properties and can help delay the skin's signs of aging. It has a gently calming effect on the nervous system and can bring peace of mind.

KEY PROPERTIES AND CHARACTERISTICS

Stimulating, highly antiseptic, expectorant, carminative, anti-inflammatory, purifying, healing, and uplifting.

BLENDS

Blends particularly well with frankincense, with which it is often linked, spice oils, cedarwood, cypress, lemon, and sandalwood.

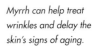

Myrrh can help treat wrinkles and delay the skin's signs of aging.

Coriander Coriandrum sativuc

The cilantro plant has been cultivated for at least 3,000 years and is widely used in Asian and Middle Eastern cookery. The essential oil—called coriander—distilled from the crushed seeds, has a sweet, spicy aroma.

Coriander oil is extracted from the crushed, ripe seeds.

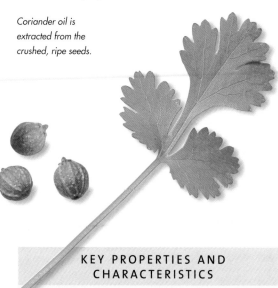

Coriander oil has warming and analgesic properties, which can help treat sprains.

USES

Coriander is an excellent digestive tonic and appetite stimulant, and is used in the treatment of anorexia, colic, diarrhea, indigestion, flatulence, and nausea. The oil's stimulatory properties are beneficial for the nervous system and for treating problems such as apathy, poor memory, and fatigue. Coriander oil has a noted effect on the circulation and as such is used to treat hemorrhoids, fluid retention, and poor circulation. Its warming and analgesic properties relieve the pain of headaches, neuralgia, rheumatism, muscular stiffness, and aches and sprains. Coriander's aphrodisiac qualities are thought to help restore libido diminished by fatigue.

KEY PROPERTIES AND CHARACTERISTICS

Stimulating, tonifying, warming, aphrodisiac, and pain-relieving.

BLENDS

Blends well with bergamot, clary sage, frankincense, jasmine, sandalwood, and other spice oils.

CORIANDER SEEDS

Cilantro leaves are widely used in Asian and Middle Eastern cookery. They give food an aromatic, sweet, spicy flavor.

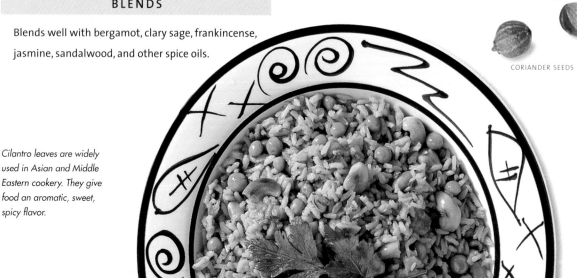

Cypress Cupressus sempervirens

The tall, evergreen cypress is native to the Mediterranean and has been used as a source of incense and for medicinal purposes for thousands of years. The oil is distilled from the leaves, cones, needles, and twigs and has a fresh, resinous odor reminiscent of pine.

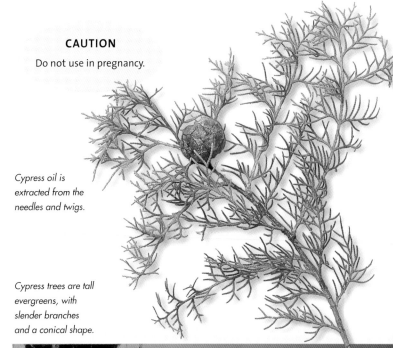

CAUTION

Do not use in pregnancy.

Cypress oil is extracted from the needles and twigs.

Cypress trees are tall evergreens, with slender branches and a conical shape.

· USES

Cypress has a tonifying and balancing effect on the female reproductive system and is used to treat period problems and alleviate the symptoms of menopause. Its effect on the circulation makes it very useful for treating varicose veins, hemorrhoids, and chilblains, and reducing fluid retention. Cypress may help to relieve muscular aches and pain and swelling of the joints. Excessive discharges such as incontinence, heavy perspiration, and nosebleeds, respond well to its astringent properties. Its antispasmodic properties relieve coughing.

KEY PROPERTIES AND CHARACTERISTICS

Detoxifying, refreshing, astringent, tonifying, antiseptic, antispasmodic, and purifying.

BLENDS

Blends well with cedarwood, clary sage, frankincense, juniper, lavender, mandarin, orange, and sandalwood.

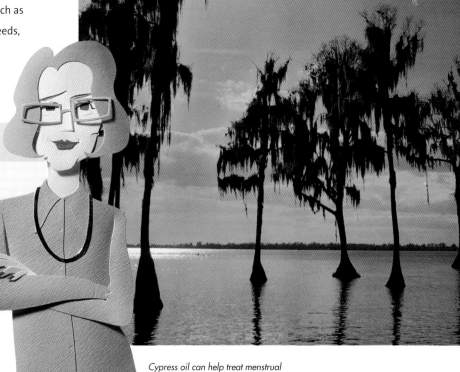

Cypress oil can help treat menstrual problems and the symptoms of menopause.

Lemongrass
Cymbopogon citratus

Lemongrass oil is extracted by steam distillation of finely chopped, partially dried leaves.

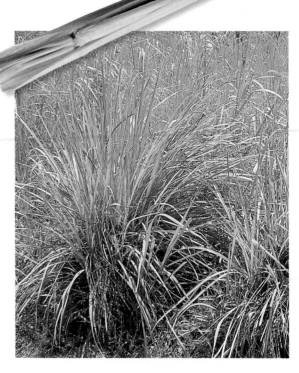

This aromatic grass has long been used as a culinary herb throughout Asia, and in Indian medicine to treat infections and reduce fever. The essential oil is distilled from finely chopped grass and has a strong, lemony aroma.

KEY PROPERTIES AND CHARACTERISTICS

Antidepressant, febrifugal, stimulant, tonifying, deodorizing, astringent, refreshing, and antiseptic.

BLENDS

Blends well with cedarwood, coriander, eucalyptus, lavender, peppermint, rosemary, thyme, and vetiver.

Lemongrass is a popular culinary herb that stimulates the appetite.

CAUTION

Do not use on babies or young children. May irritate sensitive skin.

USES

Lemongrass stimulates the appetite and may be beneficial for treating gastric infections and indigestion. It is stimulating, energizing, and a mild antidepressant, and alleviates stress-related conditions and nervous tension. Strained and aching muscles respond well to lemongrass. Its fever-reducing and antiseptic properties make it suitable for treating infections. It is a good post-illness tonic and boosts the nervous system. Lemongrass can help balance oily skin and excessive perspiration. It also makes a good insect repellent and deodorant.

Palmarosa

Cymbopogon martinii

Similar to lemongrass, palmarosa is used in Ayurvedic medicine to combat infectious diseases. The essential oil is extracted from the chopped grass and is used extensively in soap. It has a sweet, floral fragrance redolent of geranium and rose.

Palmarosa oil can help treat stress-related conditions and nervous exhaustion.

KEY PROPERTIES AND CHARACTERISTICS

Cooling, tonifying, soothing, mildly aphrodisiac, gentle antiseptic, and rejuvenating.

BLENDS

Blends well with sandalwood, cedarwood, frankincense, citrus oils, lavender, and geranium.

USES

Palmarosa has a balancing action on the skin and is best known for its use in skin care. It can help hydrate dry skin and reduce the oily secretions of greasy skin. It stimulates cell regeneration and improves the appearance of aging or tired skin. Palmarosa's antiseptic properties make it beneficial for treating acne, dermatitis, and minor skin infections. It may be used during pregnancy to help prevent stretch marks. The oil has a soothing effect on the nervous system and is useful in the treatment of stress and anxiety. It acts as a gentle tonic and aid to digestion.

Palmarosa oil is extracted from the fresh or dried grass.

This essential oil is used in many face creams and suits all skin types.

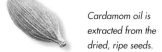

CARDAMOM SEEDS

*Cardamom oil is
extracted from the
dried, ripe seeds.*

Cardamom
Elettaria cardamomum

Cardamom has been used in Traditional Chinese Medicine and Indian Ayurvedic medicine for thousands of years, mainly for treating respiratory diseases, fevers and digestive complaints. The oil, distilled from the dried seeds, has a warm, spicy, aromatic smell.

KEY PROPERTIES AND CHARACTERISTICS

Soothing, antispasmodic, restorative, carminative, warming, diuretic, stimulating and refreshing.

BLENDS

Blends well with bergamot, frankincense, clove, ylang ylang, lemon and rose.

USES

Cardamom is mainly used as a digestive remedy to alleviate flatulence, heartburn, nausea, indigestion and colic. It acts as a general tonic for the digestive system and speeds up sluggish digestion. In India cardamom is believed to have aphrodisiac qualities and is used to reduce the feelings of stress and tension that may be inhibiting sexual fulfilment. Its restorative properties make it effective in treating physical and mental fatigue. Cardamom can be used in a mouthwash to treat bad breath. It has diuretic properties and may alleviate fluid retention and cellulite.

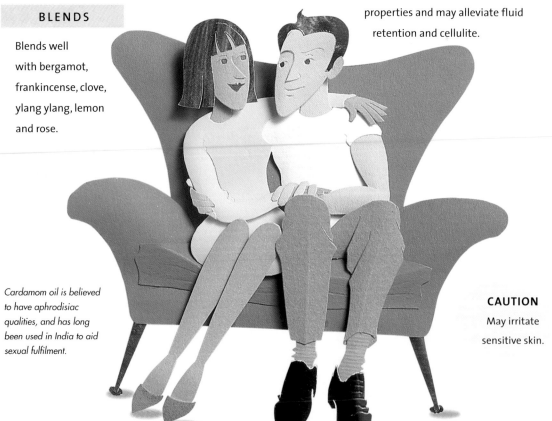

*Cardamom oil is believed
to have aphrodisiac
qualities, and has long
been used in India to aid
sexual fulfilment.*

CAUTION
May irritate sensitive skin.

Blue gum eucalyptus

Eucalyptus globulus

The blue gum eucalyptus tree is indigenous to Australia and is a medicinal herb traditionally used by the aboriginal population. The essential oil is extracted by steam distillation from the tree's leaves and twigs and it has a strong, medicinal, camphoraceous aroma.

KEY PROPERTIES AND CHARACTERISTICS

Bactericidal, antiseptic, antiviral, refreshing, warming, antibiotic, decongestant, pain relieving and anti-inflammatory.

CAUTION

Do not use with homeopathic remedies. Avoid if you have high blood pressure or epilepsy.

BLENDS

Blends particularly well with cypress, lavender, lemon, pine and rosemary.

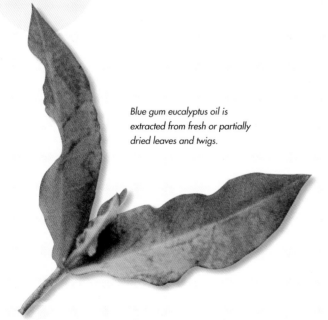

Blue gum eucalyptus oil is extracted from fresh or partially dried leaves and twigs.

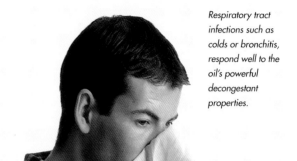

Respiratory tract infections such as colds or bronchitis, respond well to the oil's powerful decongestant properties.

USES

Eucalyptus is a powerful decongestant and is particularly good for treating respiratory tract infections such as colds, flu, sinusitis, bronchitis and pneumonia. Muscular pains and rheumatism benefit from its pain-relieving and anti-inflammatory properties. Eucalyptus has a stimulating effect and strengthens the nervous system. The oil makes an effective antiseptic room spray and insect repellent. Eucalyptus is also useful for treating insect bites, wounds, burns and blisters, and urinary tract infections respond well to it.

Fennel

Foeniculum vulgare

Fennel has long been used as a medicinal herb, and was eaten by the Romans to promote good health and prevent obesity. The essential oil, an ingredient in children's gripe water, is distilled from crushed seeds and has a spicy, peppery, aniseed smell.

Fennel has feathery leaves with an aniseed fragrance.

KEY PROPERTIES AND CHARACTERISTICS

Anti-inflammatory, detoxifying, laxative, revitalising, stimulating and diuretic.

BLENDS

Blends well with geranium, lavender, peppermint, rose and sandalwood.

FENNEL SEEDS

CAUTION

Do not use if pregnant or epileptic, and avoid using on children. Fennel is narcotic in large doses.

USES

There are two varieties of fennel: bitter and sweet. Bitter fennel is not suitable for the skin. Fennel calms and tones the digestive system and is therefore useful for treating nausea, indigestion, constipation, stomach cramps and bloating. It is an excellent detoxifier and is used as a remedy for hangovers or overeating. Its natural oestrogen content may promote weight loss, alleviate menstrual problems and menopausal disorders, and may help to stimulate breast milk production in nursing mothers. Fennel is a mild expectorant so is useful for respiratory infections.

Fennel oil is a powerful detoxifier. Use under the supervision of a qualified professional or doctor.

Hyssop Hyssopus officinalis

This ancient herb, mentioned in the Bible, has long been valued for its medicinal powers and is used to flavor liqueurs such as Chartreuse. The essential oil has a strong, spicy, grassy aroma and is distilled from the small, blue flowers and leaves.

KEY PROPERTIES AND CHARACTERISTICS

Bitter, aromatic, astringent, febrifugal, tonic, expectorant, antispasmodic and bactericidal.

BLENDS

Blends well with lavender, ylang ylang, sandalwood, citrus oils, clary sage, cypress, rosemary and geranium.

Hyssop is extracted from the lance-shaped leaves and flowering tops.

CAUTION

Do not use if pregnant or epileptic.

USES

Hyssop oil has a tonic effect on the digestive, urinary, nervous and respiratory systems. The oil is effective when treating respiratory tract infections and congestion, feverish illnesses and coughs. Hyssop acts as a general tonic for the circulation and is useful in the treatment of low blood pressure. Stress-related problems and anxieties may be relieved by its sedative and tonic properties. Hyssop promotes menstruation and is helpful in cases of scanty periods. It may accelerate the healing process of cuts and bruises.

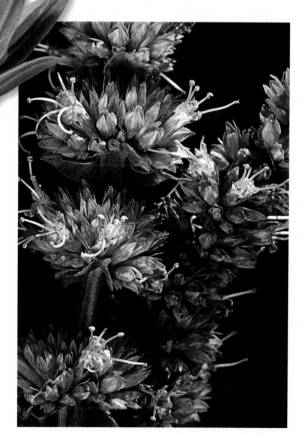

Hyssop has purple-blue flowers growing on woody stems.

Jasmine Jasminum officinale

Jasmine oil is good for hot, dry and inflamed skin and promotes the skin's elasticity.

This sturdy, evergreen, climbing shrub has long been valued for its fragrant flowers. Solvent extraction from a vast amount of flowers produces a concrete, which is then separated with alcohol to produce an absolute. Essential oil is obtained from the absolute by steam distillation, and has an intensely rich, heady, floral scent.

KEY PROPERTIES AND CHARACTERISTICS

Antidepressant, uplifting, soothing, calming, aphrodisiac and anti-inflammatory.

Jasmine oil comes from its fragrant, delicate, star-shaped flowers.

USES

Jasmine's main effect is on the emotions, and it promotes a sense of well-being, relaxation, confidence and optimism. Jasmine is a classic aphrodisiac oil because of its relaxing properties and is reputed to be beneficial for treating impotence and frigidity. It can stimulate contractions in labour and relieve pain, and helps to treat postnatal depression. Jasmine is suitable for all skin types but it is particularly beneficial for hot, dry and inflamed skin, and may maintain the skin's elasticity.

BLENDS

Blends well with bergamot, clary sage, orange, rose, sandalwood and ylang ylang.

CAUTION
Do not use in pregnancy until labour is well established.

Jasmine promotes general well-being, relaxation, confidence and optimism.

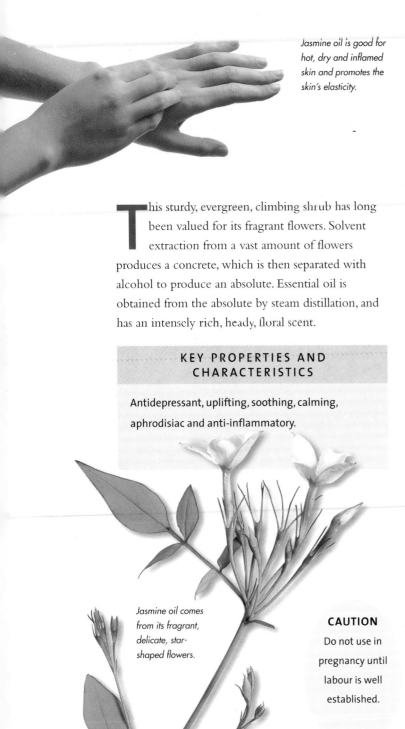

Juniper Juniperus communis

This slow-growing, evergreen shrub or vine grows up to 10m/34ft high. It produces small black berries which have been used for many years to combat disease, to flavor gin and for various culinary purposes. Juniper oil is distilled from the berries, needles and twigs, and has a fresh, peppery fragrance.

CAUTION
Avoid during pregnancy. Not suitable if you have kidney disease.

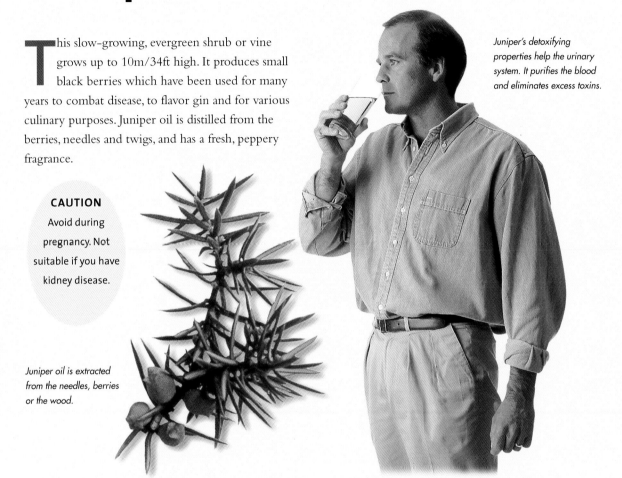

Juniper oil is extracted from the needles, berries or the wood.

Juniper's detoxifying properties help the urinary system. It purifies the blood and eliminates excess toxins.

KEY PROPERTIES AND CHARACTERISTICS

Warming, stimulating, tonifying, detoxifying, disinfectant, astringent and diuretic.

BLENDS

Blends well with bergamot, other citrus oils, cypress, sandalwood, clary sage, vetiver and rosemary.

USES

Juniper's main action is on the urinary system. Its diuretic and detoxifying properties purify the blood and encourage the elimination of uric acid and excess toxins. It relieves fluid retention and is used to treat kidney stones, rheumatism and gout, and cystitis. Juniper oil is beneficial for haemorrhoids and chilblains. Skin problems, particularly weeping eczema and acne, respond well to juniper. It helps to clear the mind and to promote self-esteem. Juniper makes an excellent disinfectant.

JUNIPER BERRIES

Lavender
Lavandula angustifolia

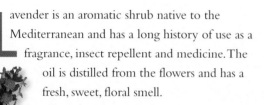

Lavender can be used neat on cuts, wounds or burns, and is a strong antiseptic.

Lavender is an aromatic shrub native to the Mediterranean and has a long history of use as a fragrance, insect repellent and medicine. The oil is distilled from the flowers and has a fresh, sweet, floral smell.

KEY PROPERTIES AND CHARACTERISTICS

Non-toxic, balancing, strong antiseptic, restorative, relaxing, analgesic, antispasmodic, bactericidal, anti-inflammatory, antidepressant.

BLENDS

Blends well with citrus oils, floral oils such as rose, geranium, ylang ylang and clove.

CAUTION
Best avoided in early pregnancy.

USES

The soothing, calming and antidepressant qualities of this versatile oil make it suitable for treating any physical symptom that is the result of stress or nervous tension. Because it is antispasmodic and a decongestant, it is effective in treating coughs, colds, flu, bronchitis and pneumonia. Its bactericidal and anti-inflammatory properties make lavender excellent for treating thrush and cystitis. Lavender is a good painkiller, suitable for treating headaches, earache, neuralgia, muscular pain and rheumatism. As a first aid remedy lavender can be used neat on cuts, wounds, burns, insect bites and stings.

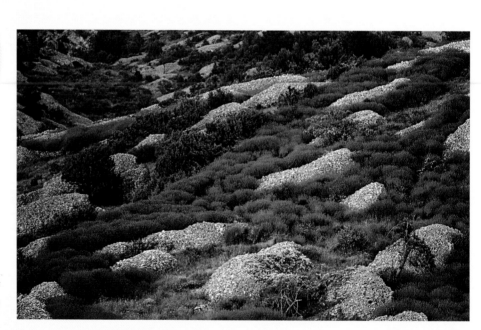

Mediterranean fields of lavender fill the air with a sweet, floral smell.

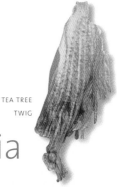

Tea tree Melaleuca alternifolia

Tea tree is an ancient remedy used by Australian aboriginals to treat infected wounds, and was included in first aid kits during the Second World War. The oil is distilled from the leaves and twigs and has a strong, fresh, camphoraceous aroma.

KEY PROPERTIES AND CHARACTERISTICS

Healing, bactericidal, anti-fungal, antiseptic, antiviral and cicatrisant.

BLENDS

Blends particularly well with other strongly antiseptic oils such as clove, eucalyptus, lavender, lemon, rosemary and pine.

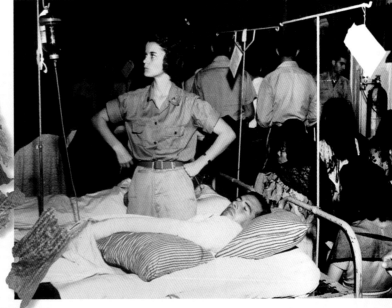

Tea tree oil was used by nurses in the Second World War for its antiseptic properties.

USES

Tea tree oil Is mainly used to combat all kinds of infection. It is effective in treating a wide range of first aid and acute ailments, and promotes the formation of scar tissue. It strengthens the immune system and promotes resistance to infection. Tea tree oil relieves the symptoms of thrush and cystitis and many other genital infections. It can be applied locally to treat such conditions as athlete's foot, ringworm, warts and verrucae, herpes, acne, burns, blisters and dandruff. It is also helpful in treating colds, fever, flu and infectious illnesses.

CAUTION
May irritate sensitive skin.

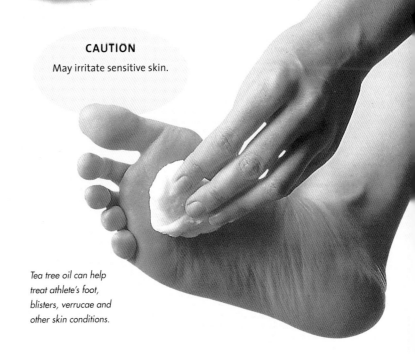

Tea tree oil can help treat athlete's foot, blisters, verrucae and other skin conditions.

Niaouli

Melaleuca viridiflora

Niaouli oil is distilled from the Melaleuca's leaves and twigs.

Also native to Australia, niaouli is closely related to tea tree, and shares its strongly antiseptic and stimulating properties. The essential oil is distilled from fresh twigs, leaves, and shoots, and has a strong, penetrating smell.

CAUTION
Dilute well, since it may irritate the skin.

USES

Niaouli is used mainly in the treatment of respiratory illnesses. It clears the respiratory tract and is very helpful for colds, catarrhal conditions, fevers, and flu. The oil stimulates the growth of new skin, helping to heal burns, treat wounds, and relieve oily skin conditions. It also stimulates the immune system, and its bactericidal properties make it good for treating cystitis and other urinary infections. In orthodox medicine, a thin layer of niaouli oil is applied to the skin during radiation treatment to protect it from burning.

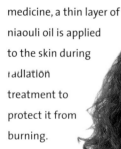

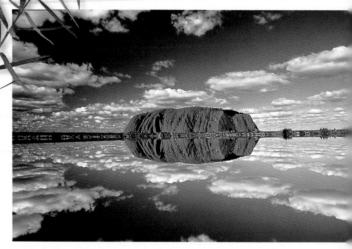

Niaouli is a variety of Melaleuca native to Australia that has similar antiseptic properties to tea tree oil.

KEY PROPERTIES AND CHARACTERISTICS

Antiseptic, bactericidal, stimulating, decongestant, fortifying, cicatrizant, and cleansing.

BLENDS

Niaouli blends particularly well with lavender, rosemary, juniper, citrus oils, and pine.

Melissa Melissa officinalis

Melissa, or lemon balm, has long been praised for its mood-lifting powers. The lemony, fresh, sweet-smelling essential oil is extracted from the leaves and flowers, but the yield is small and melissa oil is frequently adulterated with other lemon oils.

KEY PROPERTIES AND CHARACTERISTICS

Calming, uplifting, antispasmodic, cooling, and good for allergies.

USES

Traditionally known as a tonic for depression, melissa is useful for treating many nervous system problems, since it relieves anxiety, lifts the spirits, and calms hysteria. It is a tonic to the uterus, regulates menstruation, and eases painful periods. Melissa's antispasmodic properties help cases of colic, indigestion, flatulence, and nausea. It has antihistamine properties and can be beneficial for asthma sufferers and allergic skin conditions. Melissa has a calming effect on the heart, reducing palpitations and panic attacks, and is useful in cases of shock and high blood pressure.

BLENDS

Blends well with citrus oils, camomile, geranium, lavender, tea tree, and hyssop.

CAUTION
Avoid in pregnancy.
May irritate sensitive skin.

Melissa regulates menstruation and can alleviate period pain.

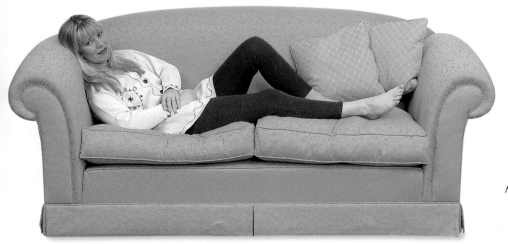

Melissa oil, or lemon balm, is extracted from the leaves and flowering tops.

Peppermint Mentha piperita

Peppermint is a herb whose characteristic smell and taste is imparted by menthol. It has been taken as a digestive remedy for thousands of years and is widely used as a flavoring. The essential oil is distilled from the flowering herb and has a fresh, minty smell.

There are hundreds of varieties of mint, which continue to hybridize and are often difficult to identify.

KEY PROPERTIES AND CHARACTERISTICS

Cooling, refreshing, stimulating, tonifying, expectorant, antiseptic, and a painkiller.

BLENDS

Blends well with lavender, rosemary, lemon, eucalyptus, sandalwood, marjoram, pine, and rosemary.

USES

Peppermint tones and settles the digestive system and is particularly useful for treating symptoms of a sluggish digestion such as flatulence and indigestion, hiccups and belching. It is a digestive antiseptic and relieves colic and gastric spasms. Peppermint is suitable for treating nausea. It refreshes and tonifies the nervous system, relieving migraine, headaches, and mental fatigue. As an expectorant, it is good for treating coughs and colds, and reduces fever and cools the body. Its pain-relieving properties alleviate toothache and headaches. Peppermint oil can help treat bad breath when used in a mouthwash. It is a useful deodorant and insect repellent.

CAUTION
May irritate sensitive skin.

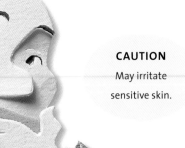

Used in mouthwash, peppermint oil can help treat bad breath.

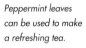

Peppermint leaves can be used to make a refreshing tea.

Myrtle Myrtus communis

This aromatic shrub has been a symbol of good luck and also used for medicinal purposes and in skin products since ancient times. Myrtle leaves are often worn in bridal headdresses. The essential oil is distilled from the twigs, leaves, and flowers, and has a fresh, violet-like scent.

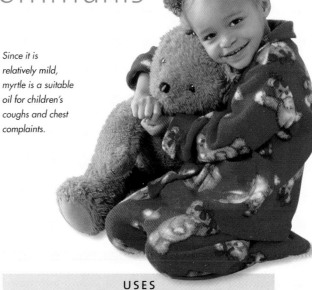

Since it is relatively mild, myrtle is a suitable oil for children's coughs and chest complaints.

KEY PROPERTIES AND CHARACTERISTICS

Antiseptic, aphrodisiac, regulating, decongestant, and mildly sedative.

BLENDS

Blends well with bergamot, ginger, rosemary, tea tree, and clary sage.

CAUTION
Prolonged use may irritate the mucous membranes.

USES

Myrtle's antiseptic and astringent qualities make it beneficial for treating skin conditions, particularly oily skin and acne. It is also used for urinary infections and may act as a tonic to the womb, and eases diarrhea and hemorrhoids. Myrtle is effective in treating respiratory conditions and, because it does not smell as strongly as eucalyptus, it can be used in a child's burner to relieve chest congestion and catarrh. Myrtle is calming, uplifting, refreshing, and soothing, good for alleviating feelings of anger and depression.

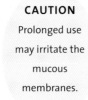

Myrtle is extracted from the leaves and twigs.

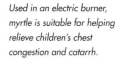

Used in an electric burner, myrtle is suitable for helping relieve children's chest congestion and catarrh.

Basil Ocimum basilicum

Basil is a popular culinary herb and an important treatment in Ayurvedic medicine for respiratory disorders. It can also be used as an antidote to snakebite. The oil is extracted from the whole plant and has an intense, pungent, clovelike odor.

Basil leaves have a strong, aromatic scent. The oil is extracted from the flowering herb.

KEY PROPERTIES AND CHARACTERISTICS

Cooling, balancing, strengthening, expectorant, restorative, uplifting, stimulating, and refreshing.

BLENDS

Blends well with lavender, bergamot, cedarwood, lemon, geranium, marjoram, and rose.

CAUTION
May irritate sensitive skin. Do not use during pregnancy.

Basil oil works well on tired muscles and has a reviving effect on the nervous system.

USES

Basil oil is an excellent nerve tonic and has a reviving, strengthening, and balancing effect on the nervous system. It relieves anxiety, nervous tension, brain fatigue, and insomnia, and can improve concentration. It works well on the digestive system, relieves stomach cramps, and is beneficial for treating gastric infections. Basil's antiseptic and expectorant properties help all types of chest infection, congested sinuses, and head colds. It is used to treat tired muscles and eases rheumatism and gout. Basil is a successful insect repellent and can be used to treat insect bites and stings.

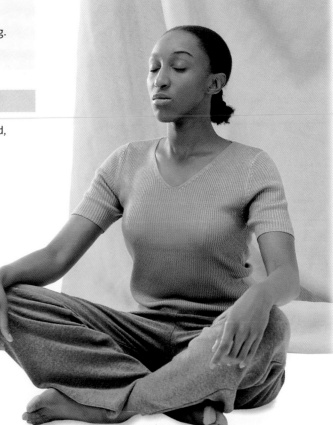

Marjoram Origanum majorana

Marjoram was a particular favorite of the Ancient Greeks, thought to bring good fortune and promote longevity. The essential oil is distilled from the dried flowering heads and leaves, and has a warm, spicy scent.

CAUTION

Best avoided during pregnancy. Not suitable for small children.

KEY PROPERTIES AND CHARACTERISTICS

Warming, relaxing, sedative, calming, pain-relieving, and antispasmodic.

Marjoram oil can help alleviate insomnia caused by nervous tension.

BLENDS

Blends well with bergamot, lavender, cypress, eucalyptus, orange, rosemary, and geranium.

USES

Marjoram oil is a tonic for the circulatory system and can be used to improve circulation and treat high blood pressure and constricted arteries. It is very effective at relieving period pains and alleviates symptoms of PMS such as irritability and anxiety. Sinus pain, headaches, and migraines, especially those caused by stress, respond well to marjoram's pain-relieving properties. It relieves colic and acts as a mild laxative. Marjoram is a sedative and alleviates insomnia and nervous tension. It is also useful for treating chest infections.

Sweet marjoram is closely related to oregano, but is less bitter. It is used in Mediterranean cooking.

Geranium

Pelargonium graveolens

Geranium oil is extracted from the fragrant flowers, leaves, and stalks of the plant.

A native of South Africa but now widely cultivated, geranium is one of the most important oils in perfumery. The essential oil is distilled from the flowers, leaves, and stems, and has a penetrating, sweet, floral smell.

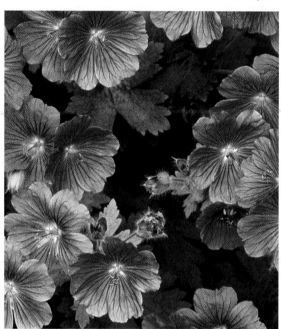

KEY PROPERTIES AND CHARACTERISTICS

Cooling, calming, uplifting, diuretic, refreshing, analgesic, and balancing.

BLENDS

Complementary oils include bergamot, lavender, rose, rosewood, sandalwood, patchouli, palmarosa, lemon, and marjoram.

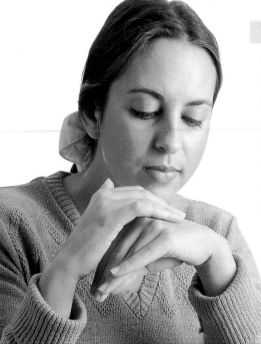

Geranium oil calms the nervous system and lifts depression, treating panic attacks and palpitations.

USES

Geranium is a balancing oil that has a calming and cooling effect on the nervous system; it is useful for treating restlessness and anxiety and lifts depression. Traditionally regarded as a feminine oil, geranium is a valuable remedy for menstrual and menopausal problems. Its calming effect makes it beneficial for treating panic attacks and palpitations. It relieves fluid retention and stimulates the flow of lymph and blood. Geranium's analgesic properties help to relieve the pain of shingles and neuralgia. Geranium oil is a popular skin care ingredient, suitable for dry or oily skin.

Scots pine Pinus sylvestris

Pines of all kinds have been used medicinally around the world since the earliest times. Pine oil is used in disinfectants, insecticides, detergents, and toiletries, and is distilled from the needles, cones, and twigs. It has a fresh, sharp smell.

USES

Pine is a powerful decongestant used to treat respiratory problems such as bronchitis, asthma, catarrh, and hay fever. It eases breathlessness and clears the sinuses. Its restorative properties and tonic effects refresh tired minds and can alleviate apathy, mental fatigue, and nervous exhaustion. Pine oil cleanses the kidneys and is beneficial for treating urinary infections such as urethritis and cystitis. It stimulates the circulation and alleviates muscular pains, rheumatism, and arthritis.

CAUTION

Check the source of your oil, as some varieties of pine are toxic. Do not use on children or the elderly.

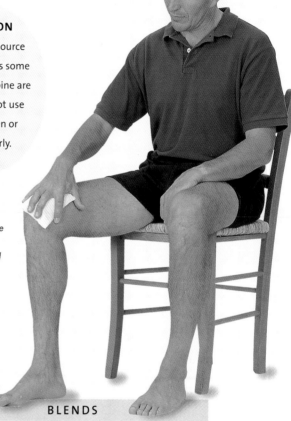

Scotch pine oil can help alleviate muscular pain, rheumatism, and arthritis.

Scotch pine oil is extracted from the needles, cones, and twigs.

BLENDS

Cedarwood, eucalyptus, cypress, lavender, rosemary, and tea tree oils are good for blending.

KEY PROPERTIES AND CHARACTERISTICS

Refreshing, invigorating, antiseptic, decongestant, stimulant, diuretic, expectorant, deodorizing, insecticidal.

Black pepper Piper nigrum

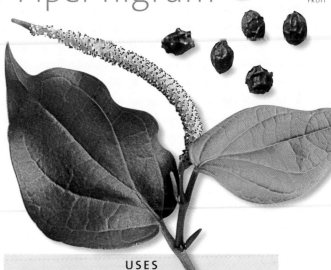

PEPPER
FRUIT

The dried whole fruit of the pepper plant, a vinelike shrub, has been used in China and India for thousands of years in cooking and as a medicine. The essential oil is extracted from dried, crushed peppercorns and has a spicy, warm aroma.

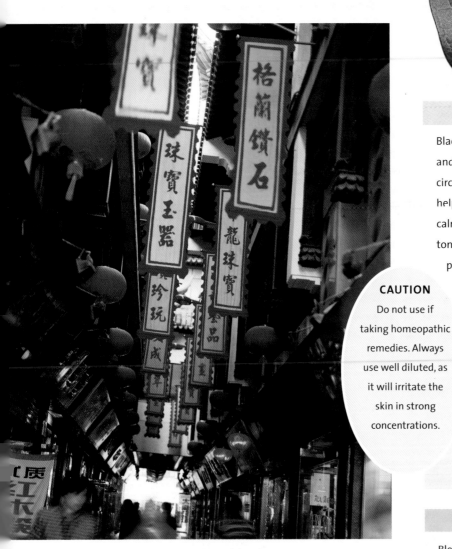

Black pepper has been used in China as a culinary spice for thousands of years. The oil is extracted from the black peppercorns, dried and crushed.

USES

Black pepper stimulates the circulatory, digestive, and nervous systems and can be used to treat poor circulation, sluggish digestion, and fatigue. It is helpful in treating a range of digestive disorders, calming the stomach, stimulating the appetite, and toning the muscles of the intestines. It alleviates painful joints and muscular aches and pains. Its warming properties make it beneficial for treating respiratory conditions, and as an expectorant it helps to clear catarrh.

CAUTION

Do not use if taking homeopathic remedies. Always use well diluted, as it will irritate the skin in strong concentrations.

KEY PROPERTIES AND CHARACTERISTICS

Aphrodisiac, warming, stimulant, laxative, tonifying, detoxifying, and restorative.

BLENDS

Blends well with lavender, spice oils, frankincense, lemon, and marjoram.

Patchouli Pogostemon cablin

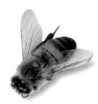

This large-leaved herb, native to tropical Asia, is a renowned antidote to insect and snake bites and has long been a popular ingredient in perfume. The leaves are lightly fermented to break down the cell walls and then steam-distilled to produce the essential oil. The oil has a very distinctive, intense, musky, exotic fragrance which is not to everyone's taste.

KEY PROPERTIES AND CHARACTERISTICS

Antidepressant, aphrodisiac, astringent, cicatrizant, stimulating, diuretic, deodorizing, and antimicrobal.

USES

Patchouli is effective in the treatment of acne, oily skin, dermatitis, dandruff, and fungal infections of the skin. It promotes cell regeneration, making it beneficial for wrinkles and aging skin, and it can help the formation of scar tissue and aid wound-healing. It is helpful for treating cellulite and water retention. Patchouli is an antidepressant, is thought to restore libido, and has a profound effect on the nervous system. It can be sedative if used in large quantities.

Patchouli oil is extracted from the fragrant, furry leaves. It is useful for treating bee stings.

BLENDS

Cedarwood, geranium, lavender, rose, bergamot, and sandalwood.

Patchouli oil can help to treat dandruff when used in a shampoo.

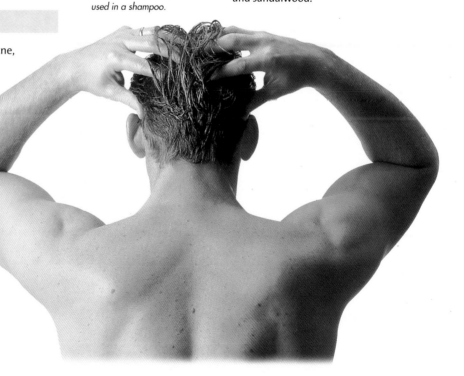

Rose Rosa centifolia, R. damascena

The rose was probably the first plant to be distilled by the Persian physician Avicenna. Rose oil is usually produced from the petals of two types of rose, the cabbage and damask rose. The oil has a deep, rich, sweet, floral scent.

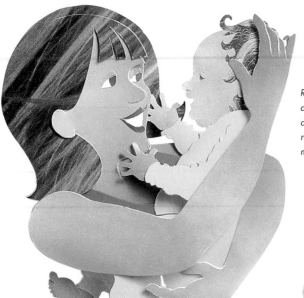

Rose oil can help alleviate postnatal depression and regulate the menstrual cycle.

USES

Rose oil increases feelings of vitality and lifts the mood. A wide range of stress-related conditions respond well to rose oil and it acts as a mild sedative and antidepressant, useful in times of shock and melancholy. It is a well-known aphrodisiac. Rose has an affinity with the female reproductive system, and is used to treat infertility and frigidity, alleviate PMS and postnatal depression, and regulate the menstrual cycle. It relieves digestive spasms, nausea, and constipation, has a detoxifying effect, and rejuvenates and heals the skin.

Rose oil is extracted from the fresh petals. It has a deep, sweet, floral scent.

KEY PROPERTIES AND CHARACTERISTICS

Antidepressant, aphrodisiac, relaxing, strengthening, detoxifying, and uplifting.

BLENDS

Most oils, especially clary sage, lavender, patchouli, sandalwood, ylang ylang, and bergamot.

CAUTION

Do not take during the first three months of pregnancy.

Rosemary

Rosmarinus officinalis

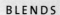
Rosemary oil is extracted from the flowering tops and leaves of the herb.

This classic culinary herb, used in the ancient world for medicinal purposes, was worn in a pouch round the neck during the Middle Ages to ward off the plague. The oil is distilled from the flowers and leaves, and has a strong, fresh, camphoraceous fragrance.

CAUTION

Do not use if pregnant, epileptic, or if you have high blood pressure.

KEY PROPERTIES AND CHARACTERISTICS

Stimulating, warming, strengthening, restorative, reviving, analgesic, purifying, and invigorating.

BLENDS

Combines well with lemongrass, basil, peppermint, and spice oils.

USES

Rosemary oil increases the circulation of blood and stimulates the nervous system, improving memory, mental alertness, and concentration. It is excellent for low blood pressure, muscular aches and pains, and helps clear headaches and migraines. Rosemary is cleansing and tonifying, good for the skin, gallbladder, and liver, and helps alleviate water retention and cellulite. It is beneficial for greasy hair and skin, dandruff, and varicose veins (but do not massage directly on or below varicose veins). It reduces digestive spasm and relieves painful periods.

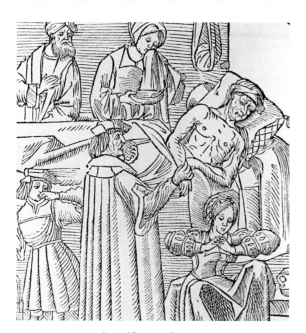
In the Middle Ages, the aromatic odor of rosemary oil helped mask the smell of the sickroom.

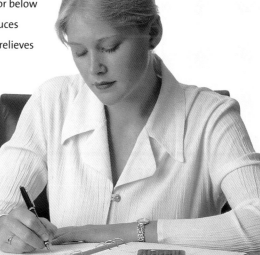
Rosemary improves mental alertness— useful when studying hard for an exam.

Clary sage Salvia sclarea

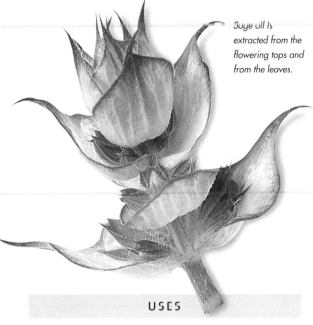

Sage oil is extracted from the flowering tops and from the leaves.

Clary sage was a popular remedy for eye problems in the Middle Ages. It is still used as a flavoring in Rhine wines. The essential oil has a strong, nutty smell and is extracted from the flowers and leaves.

KEY PROPERTIES AND CHARACTERISTICS

Relaxing, rejuvenating, revitalizing, antidepressant, sedative, tonifying, relaxing, and a uterine tonic.

BLENDS

Blends well with frankincense, cedarwood, lavender, citrus oils, and coriander.

CAUTION

Do not use in pregnancy until labor is well established. Do not take alcohol before or after use. May cause drowsiness and nightmares. Make sure you buy clary sage rather than common sage oil as it is safer to use.

USES

Clary sage has an affinity with the female reproductive system and is of great benefit for PMS and the menopause. It can ease labor pains and strengthen contractions. It is considered to be an aphrodisiac, particularly in cases of stress-related frigidity or impotence. It has become a noted antidepressant, and is excellent for elevating mood and treating a range of stress-related disorders. Clary sage relaxes muscles, is an effective pain-reliever, and benefits the digestive system.

Clary sage oil helps to elevate mood and can treat a range of stress-related disorders, migraine, and nervous tension.

Sandalwood Santalum album

Sandalwood is an important remedy in Ayurvedic and Traditional Chinese Medicine, and the finest oil comes from India. The oil has a deep, sweet, woody, exotic aroma and is distilled from the heartwood of the tree and its dried, powdered roots.

KEY PROPERTIES AND CHARACTERISTICS

Aphrodisiac, uplifting, warming, relaxing, purifying, antidepressant, and soothing.

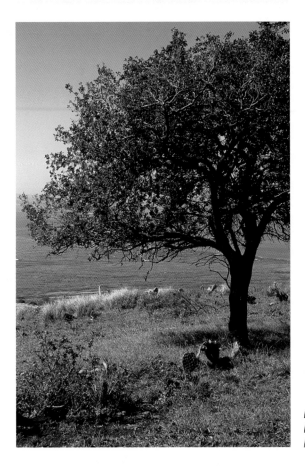

Evergreen sandalwood trees take at least 30 years to develop sufficient heartwood for oil extraction.

USES

Sandalwood is a renowned aphrodisiac, particularly for men. It has a profound effect on emotional problems, calming the nervous system and alleviating depression, and was traditionally used as an aid to meditation. It is very effective for urinary disorders, particularly cystitis and venereal infections. Sandalwood's emollient and anti-inflammatory properties soothe itching, inflamed, and dry skin, including shaving rash, and can help with dandruff. It is beneficial for respiratory tract infections such as bronchitis and sore throats. Sandalwood calms the digestive system and is appropriate for hot and painful digestive disorders such as diarrhea.

BLENDS

Suitable oils for blending include rose, jasmine, bergamot, lavender, ylang ylang, and patchouli.

Sandalwood is an aphrodisiac, especially for men. It can also help soothe inflamed skin, including shaving rash.

Clove Syzygium aromaticum

Clove trees are slender evergreens that have been cultivated in Europe for nearly 2,000 years for their culinary and medicinal properties. The flowers are popular deodorizers used in pot-pourri and pomanders. The oil is extracted from the dried flower buds and has a strong, fresh, spicy aroma.

Cloves pushed into an orange make a fragrant pomander, which can be suspended from a ribbon.

KEY PROPERTIES AND CHARACTERISTICS

Pain-relieving, stimulating, insecticide, strongly antiseptic, warming, deodorizing, antispasmodic, and carminative.

BLENDS

Blends well with other strongly antiseptic oils such as bergamot, eucalyptus, lavender, and thyme.

USES

This spicy, warming herb is a well-known pain-reliever, commonly used for treating toothache. It is also beneficial in the treatment of rheumatism, arthritis, and muscular aches and pains in general. Clove oil helps to strengthen the immune system and is a good treatment for colds and flu. Its antispasmodic and carminative properties help relieve indigestion and flatulence. Clove oil is a powerful antiseptic. It promotes the formation of scar tissue, helping combat infections and heal wounds. It is also a useful insect repellent.

CAUTION

Can cause uterine contractions so avoid in pregnancy. Not suitable for infants.

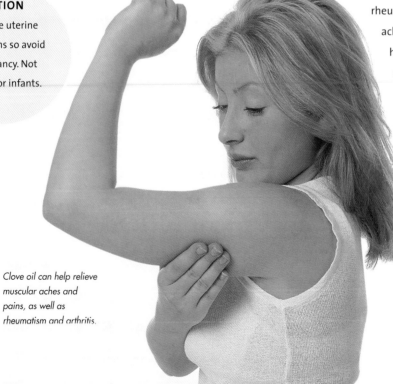

Clove oil can help relieve muscular aches and pains, as well as rheumatism and arthritis.

Thyme *Thymus vulgaris*

Used by the ancient Egyptians in the embalming process, thyme has long been valued for its culinary and healing properties and is rich in thymol, a powerful antiseptic. The flowering tops and leaves are distilled to produce the oil, which has a fresh, herbaceous scent.

KEY PROPERTIES AND CHARACTERISTICS

Antiseptic, germicide, stimulating, warming, expectorant, restorative, reviving, and purifying.

BLENDS

Blends well with other strongly antiseptic oils such as lavender, lemon, pine, clove, or tea tree.

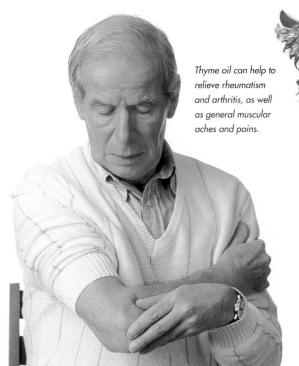

Thyme oil can help to relieve rheumatism and arthritis, as well as general muscular aches and pains.

CAUTION

Do not use if pregnant. May cause an allergic reaction on sensitive skin: dilute well. Not suitable for infants.

USES

Thyme oil acts as a general nerve tonic and is invaluable for treating all kinds of infections, particularly those of the respiratory, digestive, and urinary systems. It stimulates the production of white blood cells and helps to strengthen the immune system. Rheumatism and arthritis respond well to thyme oil. It can be used to treat low blood pressure and may be helpful for anemia. Thyme oil heals infections, sores, and boils.

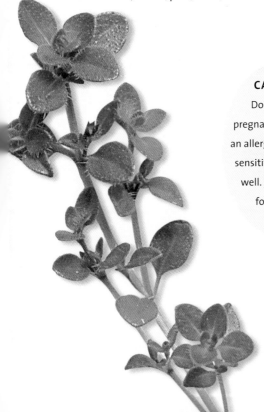

Thyme oil is extracted from the fresh, or partially dried, leaves and flowering tops.

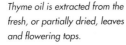

Vetiver Vetiveria zizanoides

Native to India, the vetiver plant's dense roots help prevent soil erosion during the rainy season. The oil, in great demand as a perfumery base note, is extracted from the chopped roots and has a sweet, heavy, earthy, woody aroma.

KEY PROPERTIES AND CHARACTERISTICS

Soothing, sedative, grounding, stimulating, rejuvenating, uplifting, and protective.

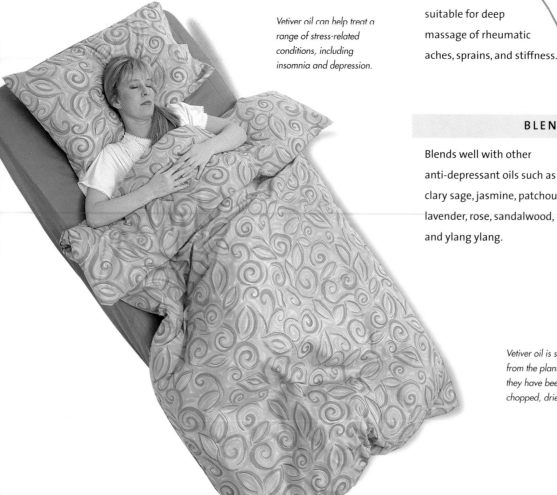

Vetiver oil can help treat a range of stress-related conditions, including insomnia and depression.

USES

This deeply relaxing oil is used mostly for its effects on the nervous system. Its tranquilizing properties render it suitable for dealing with a wide range of stress-related conditions, including insomnia and depression. Vetiver stimulates the production of red blood cells and is beneficial for anemia. In skin care, vetiver may be used to treat acne, oily skin, and sores. Vetiver promotes skin regeneration and improves the appearance of scars and wrinkles. Vetiver's pain-relieving properties make it suitable for deep massage of rheumatic aches, sprains, and stiffness.

BLENDS

Blends well with other anti-depressant oils such as clary sage, jasmine, patchouli, lavender, rose, sandalwood, and ylang ylang.

Vetiver oil is steam distilled from the plant's roots, after they have been washed, chopped, dried, and soaked.

Ginger Zingiber officinale

Ginger has been used in cooking and medicine for thousands of years, particularly in China, where it is a noted aphrodisiac. The essential oil is distilled from the roots and has a hot, spicy, pungent, sweet smell.

KEY PROPERTIES AND CHARACTERISTICS

Tonifying, stimulating, warming, pain-relieving, febrifugal, apéritif, and aphrodisiac.

CAUTION

May irritate sensitive skin.

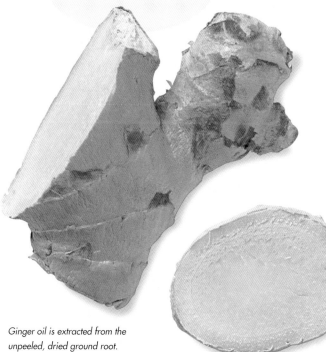

Ginger oil is extracted from the unpeeled, dried ground root.

USES

Ginger settles the digestive system and stimulates the appetite. It works well in relieving flatulence, diarrhea, nausea (including morning sickness), and indigestion. It has a major effect on the lungs, encouraging the body to throw off fevers, and acts as an expectorant. It is very effective when treating flu, chronic colds, and catarrh. Ginger strengthens the immune system and improves vitality. Ginger is a rubefacient and eases the symptoms of arthritis, rheumatism, and muscle pain. It stimulates the circulation and may alleviate varicose veins and chilblains. Ginger is a powerful nerve tonic, sharpening the senses and dispelling feelings of tiredness.

Ginger has a long history of use in Chinese cooking. It stimulates the appetite and settles the digestive system.

BLENDS

Blends well with cedarwood, rose, vetiver, patchouli, frankincense, citrus oils, and sandalwood.

Common **ailments**

This section describes a range of disorders
and lists some of the essential oils that are
commonly used to treat them. Many oils
have been used successfully for thousands
of years, and are still popular because they
are effective. Always dilute oils in a suitable
carrier when applying to the skin unless
instructed to use them neat. Be aware of
any cautions listed when using an oil and
do not hesitate to consult your doctor if you
are concerned about any condition.

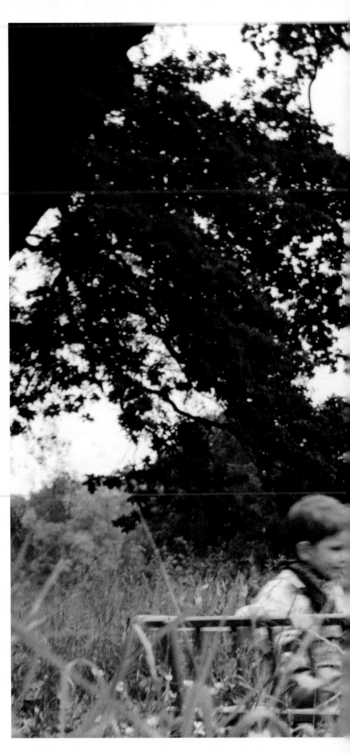

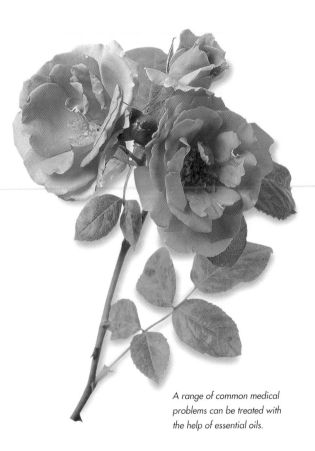

*A range of common medical
problems can be treated with
the help of essential oils.*

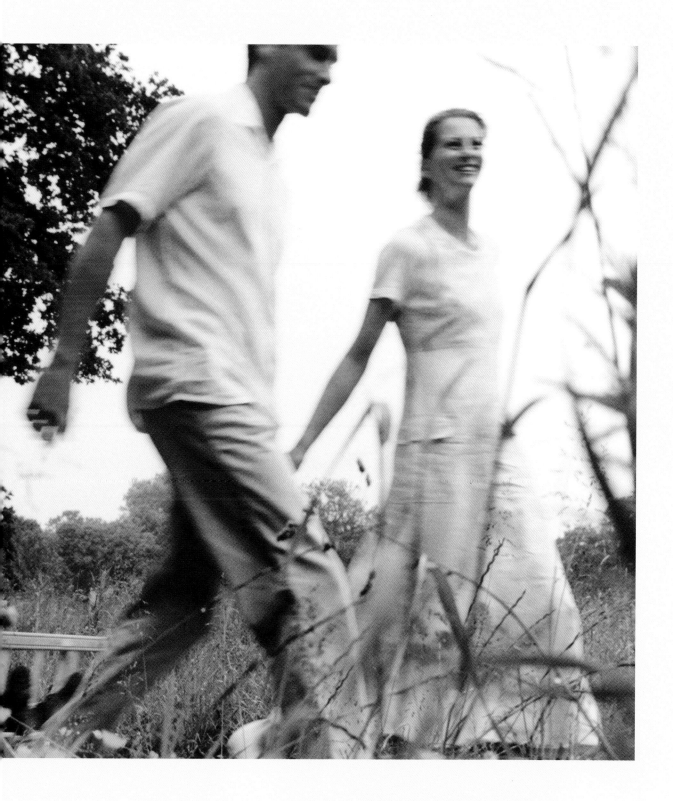

YLANG YLANG

Mind, emotions, and **nerves**

The body and the mind are closely interrelated, and many physical disorders may be rooted in problems of the mind and emotions. The central nervous system – the brain and spinal cord – is the center of our thoughts, feelings, and senses, and co-ordinates movement and all bodily processes. Essential oils are extremely beneficial as antidepressants, as they ease physical tension and engender feelings of relaxation and peace to calm the mind and body.

ANXIETY

Anxiety is a normal response to certain situations, but sometimes becomes so intense that it interferes with normal life. Anxiety may manifest as digestive disturbances, panic attacks, palpitations, poor concentration, irritability, tiredness, depression, insomnia, headaches, and back pain. Bergamot, lavender, and geranium alleviate intense anxiety, particularly when used in combination as a bath oil. Frankincense, Roman camomile, ylang ylang, melissa, and jasmine are relaxing.

DEPRESSION

Symptoms of depression include mood swings, disturbed sleep and appetite, loss of sex drive, tiredness, and aches and pains. Suitable oils to elevate mood and relieve physical symptoms include cinnamon leaf, bergamot, lavender, clary sage, neroli, camomile, ylang ylang, melissa, jasmine, cedarwood, myrtle, rose, vetiver, and geranium, which can be used in a burner, in the bath, and in massage.

Rosemary can alleviate headaches, nervous exhaustion, and stress-related disorders.

ROSEMARY

APPETITE

Depression and anxiety are often symptoms of poor eating habits, and uplifting and relaxing essential oils, such as lavender, clary sage, bergamot, neroli, and ylang ylang, may improve your mood. In cases of poor appetite due to stress, coriander acts as an stimulant. Use the oils in a vaporizer or add a few drops to bathwater.

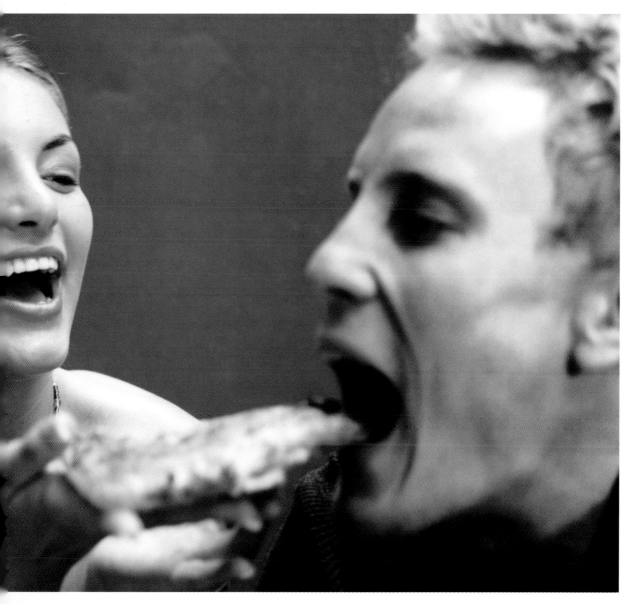

*Coriander and lemongrass stimulate the appetite,
so they are useful for treating simple loss of
appetite caused by stress.*

CHAMOMILE

HEADACHE AND MIGRAINE

Try a cool compress of lavender or peppermint, or an inhalation, massage, or bath with camomile, angelica, rosewood, marjoram, ylang ylang, melissa, or rosemary oils to relieve pain.

INSOMNIA

Disturbed sleep patterns are often caused by stress and anxiety, and quickly lead to overtiredness, mood swings, and irritability. A gentle massage before bedtime with bergamot, cypress, geranium, jasmine, basil, melissa, rose, neroli, sandalwood, or ylang ylang may promote relaxation and restful sleep, or add a few drops to bathwater or a vaporizer.

For restless children, place a few drops of lavender oil on their pillow or pajamas. Scenting the sheets with lavender oil or a few drops into the bathtub will soon help overactive or irritable children to drop off.

NEURALGIA

This pain arises from an inflamed or damaged nerve and can vary from a slight tingle to agony. The pain can be sited where the nerve reaches the skin, or can run along the length of a nerve. A compress of rosemary will improve circulation and promote healing. Camomile, eucalyptus, and lavender used in a massage oil on the affected area will relieve pain, if it is combined with rest and relaxation to heal the underlying cause.

Camomile is an effective painkiller that eases neuralgia, muscular pain, sprains, and rheumatism.

SEASONAL AFFECTIVE DISORDER

Seasonal Affective Disorder (SAD) is a type of depression brought on by lack of daylight in winter. Symptoms include lethargy, loss of libido, mood swings, sleep disorders, depression, irritability, and food cravings. A massage with uplifting and relaxing oils such as rose, lavender, neroli, or ylang ylang will improve well-being and relaxation.

STRESS

Essential oils can be very powerful in alleviating the problems caused by a modern, stressful lifestyle. Many oils work on the nervous system to relax and soothe; the best include basil, camomile, geranium, lavender, melissa, neroli, rose, bergamot, marjoram, and jasmine. Using essential oils in a massage is particularly soothing, though burning them in a vaporizer or adding to bathwater is also relaxing.

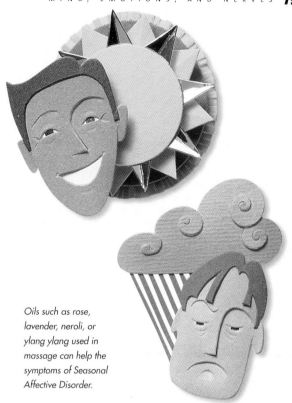

Oils such as rose, lavender, neroli, or ylang ylang used in massage can help the symptoms of Seasonal Affective Disorder.

Hair and skin

Essential oils, mixed in carrier oils, can be very effective in correcting imbalances that occur in the hair and skin.

Cedarwood, lavender, rosemary, and ylang ylang massaged into the scalp may stimulate hair growth.

DRY OR GREASY HAIR

For dry hair, try a shampoo that includes camomile (blonde), lavender, or rosemary (dark hair). For greasy hair, try cypress, rosemary, clary sage, geranium, lemon, lavender, or tea tree oil. Massage the oil into the scalp and then rinse off.

DANDRUFF

Massage a few drops of the following into the scalp to reduce flaking: cedarwood, rosemary, geranium, lavender, tea tree, or patchouli. Leave for half an hour, then rinse off. To treat cradle cap in infants, massage lavender or lemon into the scalp before bedtime and leave overnight.

HAIR LOSS

Massage cedarwood, lavender, rosemary, ylang ylang, or clary sage into the scalp to stimulate growth following temporary baldness that results from illness. Leave for half an hour, then rinse off.

Aromatic hair tonics can help to balance sebum levels and promote hair growth.

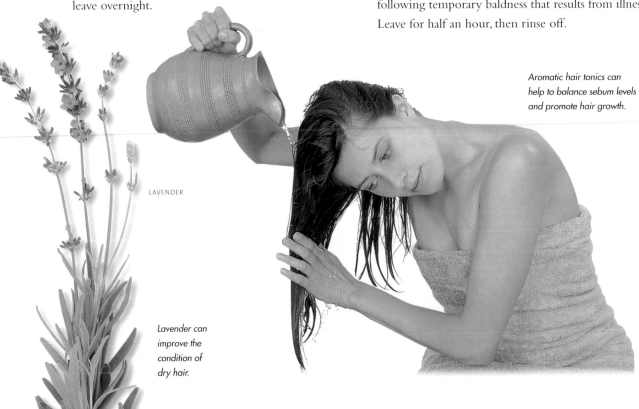

LAVENDER

Lavender can improve the condition of dry hair.

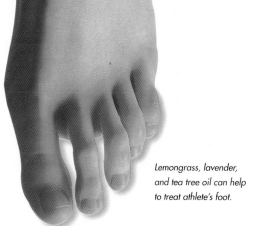

OILY SKIN AND ACNE

Many oils are healing and balancing: bergamot, palmarosa, tea tree, cedarwood, lavender, camomile, and citrus oils are particularly effective. Use in a vaporizer, in compresses, or in the bath, or steam your face over a basin of very hot water.

DRY SKIN

Cedarwood, rose, sandalwood, geranium, and palmarosa moisturize dry skin; jasmine, lavender, and camomile can be used on sensitive skin. Add to bathwater, or use as ointments or in steam treatments.

Lemongrass, lavender, and tea tree oil can help to treat athlete's foot.

ATHLETE'S FOOT

This fungal infection responds well to lemongrass, lavender, tea tree, cypress, peppermint, or black pepper oils used in a foot bath or compress.

VERRUCAS AND WARTS

Dab neat lemon or tea tree oil directly on to warts and verrucas.

WRINKLES

Several essential oils have rejuvenating properties and can improve the appearance of mature, wrinkled skin. Cypress, frankincense, clary sage, vetiver, rosewood, sandalwood, patchouli, and jasmine are noted for their cosmetic effects. Use in the bath, in ointments, or in steam treatments.

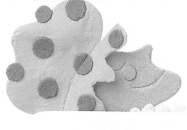

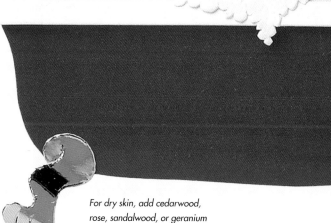

For dry skin, add cedarwood, rose, sandalwood, or geranium oil to bathwater.

Many aromatic herbs can be cultivated in your garden.

DERMATITIS, ECZEMA, AND PSORIASIS

Essential oils can help relieve the itchiness and inflammation of irritated skin, psoriasis, and other skin conditions. Lavender, bergamot, camomile, or geranium added to bathwater, or used in an ointment, are particularly beneficial.

Respiratory system

Essential oils are particularly beneficial for treating respiratory disorders. When oils are inhaled, their particles can help to clear blocked airways as they travel toward the lungs. Certain essential oils can clear excess mucus from the body, reduce fever, fight infection, and ease muscular spasms that cause breathing difficulties. Use steam inhalations with care if you have asthma.

RESPIRATORY SYSTEM

The respiratory system enables oxygen to be taken into the body
to provide the energy needed for life

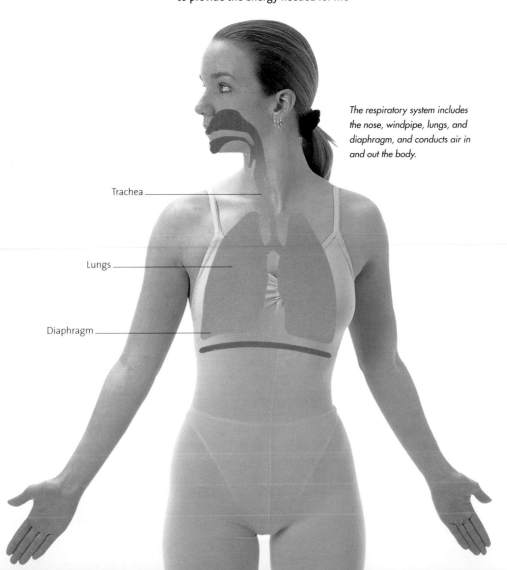

The respiratory system includes the nose, windpipe, lungs, and diaphragm, and conducts air in and out the body.

Trachea

Lungs

Diaphragm

Asthmatics can be helped by angelica, cypress, rosewood, and fennel, either in a burner or bath, or as a chest rub.

ASTHMA

Intermittent muscular spasms in the airways in the lungs cause shortness of breath, coughing, and wheezing. Use the following in a burner, in the bath, or as a chest rub to alleviate breathing difficulties: angelica, cypress, rosewood, fennel, cedarwood, bergamot, lavender, jasmine, eucalyptus, frankincense, Scots pine, lemon.

BRONCHITIS

Use the following oils in chest rubs, or add to bathwater, burn in a vaporizer, or use in an inhalation: eucalyptus, ginger, and thyme (to clear congestion); juniper, rosemary, and myrrh (to detoxify); lavender (to relax muscles).

CATARRH

The overproduction of mucus is usually caused by inflamed mucous membranes, triggered by infections such as colds and flu and by allergies. A few drops of eucalyptus, lemon, niaouli, myrtle, or cedarwood oil added to bathwater may relieve congestion.

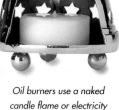

Oil burners use a naked candle flame or electricity for heat.

COLDS AND FLU

Colds and flu are caused by viruses, and symptoms include sneezing, sore throats, coughs, fever, sweating, tiredness, and headaches. Treatment focuses on relieving symptoms and building up the immune system. Try yarrow, angelica, cedarwood, cinnamon leaf, eucalyptus, niaouli, myrtle, Scots pine, tea tree, cypress, rosemary, fennel, lavender, rosewood, sandalwood, ginger, peppermint, lemon/lime, or myrrh. Use in the bath or as a chest rub.

HAYFEVER

Use the following in the bath or in a vaporizer to alleviate symptoms: ginger, lavender, basil, melissa, myrrh, and eucalyptus.

SINUSITIS

The sinuses are cavities in the facial bones that surround and are joined to the nasal cavity. Blocked sinuses can cause severe pain in the cheekbones, forehead, and upper jaw. To fight infection and clear blocked passages, try a steam inhalation with lavender, eucalyptus, myrtle, tea tree, or niaouli oil.

Those who suffer from hayfever can use ginger, lavender, and other oils in the bath or a vaporizer to help alleviate symtoms.

Essential oils can relieve the symptoms of colds and flu, as well as help build up the immune system.

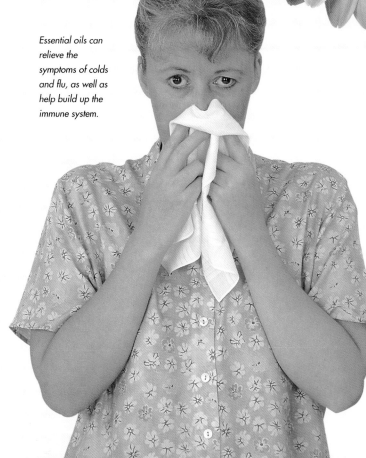

Orange oil can be used to treat palpitations, obesity, and water retention.

Circulatory system

The circulatory system consists of the blood, which transports oxygen and nutrients around the body and carbon dioxide to the lungs, and also lymph, which removes toxins and waste products, and circulates antibodies and white blood cells to counter diseases. Many essential oils have positive effects on circulation and their diuretic properties help to eliminate toxins.

CIRCULATORY SYSTEM

The heart and blood vessels circulate blood around the body, providing the tissues with oxygen and nutrients, and removing waste products.

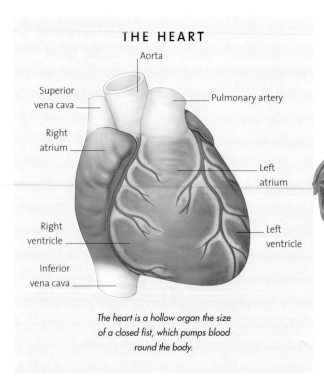

THE HEART

Aorta

Superior vena cava

Pulmonary artery

Right atrium

Left atrium

Right ventricle

Left ventricle

Inferior vena cava

The heart is a hollow organ the size of a closed fist, which pumps blood round the body.

Deoxygenated blood

Oxygenated blood

Blood is pumped around the body through a network of arteries and viens.

ANEMIA

Anemia is a deficiency in the blood of the oxygen-carrying pigment hemoglobin. It is usually caused by iron deficiency resulting from excessive blood loss, and is also common in pregnancy. Symptoms include fatigue, pallor, breathlessness, and lowered resistance to infection. A massage with Roman camomile or lavender oil may alleviate dizzy spells and palpitations associated with anemia.

BLOOD PRESSURE

Regular massages with lavender, neroli, marjoram, and ylang ylang are effective for high blood pressure. Massage with lemon, clary sage, hyssop, rosemary, or black pepper to treat low blood pressure.

PALPITATIONS

Add marjoram, lavender, mandarin, and ylang ylang to bathwater to calm palpitations caused by stress and anxiety.

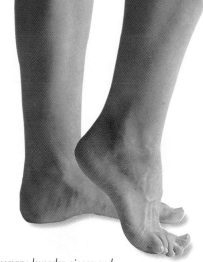

Rosemary, lavender, ginger, and juniper oil all help improve circulation and can treat varicose veins.

SWOLLEN VEINS

Poor circulation, caused by lack of exercise, standing for long periods, obesity, poor nutrition, and a sedentary lifestyle, can result in distended veins. Be very gentle when treating them and do not apply direct pressure. For varicose veins, most commonly found in the legs, massage rosemary, lavender, ginger, or juniper oil into the legs or add to the bathwater. Hemorrhoids are varicose veins around the anus, which can occur during pregnancy but are usually a consequence of chronic constipation. Relieve with compresses or baths of the following: frankincense, geranium, myrtle, rosemary, cypress, bergamot. Chilblains, red itchy swellings on the fingers and toes, can develop in cold weather. They respond well to baths with ginger, basil, juniper, lemon, rosemary, eucalyptus, and cypress, or a camomile compress.

WATER RETENTION/CELLULITE

A build-up of toxins in the tissues causes cellulite and water retention. Ease symptoms by adding the following to the bath: yarrow, juniper, geranium, orange, lemon, grapefruit, rosemary, fennel, cedarwood, cypress, lavender, angelica, and niaouli.

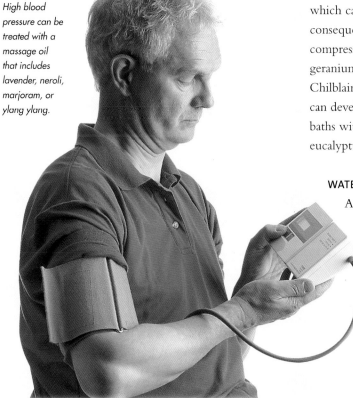

High blood pressure can be treated with a massage oil that includes lavender, neroli, marjoram, or ylang ylang.

Rosemary can help eliminate the build up of toxins that go toward causing cellulite.

Muscles, bones, and joints

Musculo-skeletal pain can affect many parts of the body. Essential oils ease muscle tension and promote the elimination of toxins that may be contributing to conditions such as rheumatism. Many oils reduce inflammation, relieve pain, and promote the healing process.

EUCALYPTUS

ARTHRITIS AND RHEUMATISM

Add to bathwater or massage with yarrow, pine, cedarwood, cinnamon leaf, lime/lemon, or juniper to reduce swelling or with black pepper, basil, marjoram, clove, thyme, or eucalyptus to stimulate the circulation. A massage or compress of lavender, vetiver, camomile, yarrow, ginger, cardamom, or rosemary will relieve pain and stiffness.

BACKACHE

Use the following oils in the bath, in a massage or in a burner to relax, relieve pain, and reduce inflammation: lavender, clary sage, blue gum eucalyptus, Scots pine, marjoram, vetiver, Roman camomile, juniper, rosemary, and basil.

CRAMP

Painful muscle spasms can affect the feet and legs, arms, hands, and stomach. Try the following in a massage oil or compress, use in a burner, or add to bathwater: lavender, geranium, melissa, camomile, marjoram, vetiver, jasmine, and ylang ylang.

MUSCLES AND BONES

Muscles and bones protect the internal organs and enable mobility.

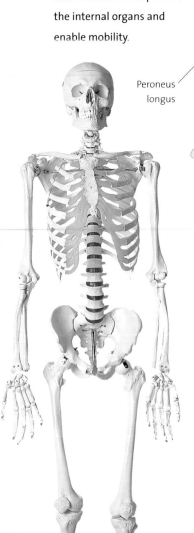

Rectus femoris

Peroneus longus

Muscles are attached to the skeleton and enable the body to move. Muscular pain is eased by essential oils.

More than 200 bones form the skeleton, the body's framework. Skeletal pain responds well to essential oils.

Digestive system

A healthy digestion is crucial for physical and emotional well-being. Digestive problems can be caused by stress and emotional disturbances, allergies, infections, or a poor diet. The following oils may improve the general tone of the digestive tract, relieve pain, and soothe muscular spasms. Use in the bath, massage, in a compress applied to the abdomen, or vaporizer.

The use of essential oils, together with a healthy diet, can help the digestive system.

DIGESTIVE SYSTEM

The digestive system processes food so that nutrients can be absorbed into the bloodstream.

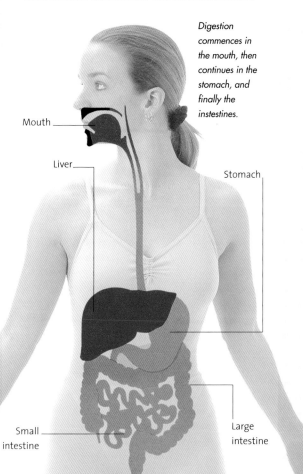

Digestion commences in the mouth, then continues in the stomach, and finally the instestines.

Mouth

Liver

Stomach

Small intestine

Large intestine

NAUSEA AND VOMITING

Angelica, ginger, fennel, peppermint, and camomile will ease nausea and settle the stomach.

INDIGESTION

Suitable oils include yarrow, angelica, coriander, frankincense, ginger, lavender, lime, camomile, rose, rosemary, basil, fennel, and cardamom.

FLATULENCE

Ease abdominal pains and bloating with a massage of yarrow, cinnamon leaf, cardamom, coriander, ginger, peppermint, or clove oil.

CONSTIPATION

Massage a few drops of the following into the abdominal region: camomile, basil, rosemary, mandarin, marjoram, fennel, ginger, or juniper.

DIARRHEA

Yarrow, camomile, sandalwood, fennel, basil, myrtle, marjoram, or ginger will ease symptoms.

LIVER COMPLAINTS

Camomile, cypress, grapefruit, juniper, lemon, and orange work as a tonic on the liver and are suitable for relieving symptoms of hepatitis and cirrhosis.

BERGAMOT
LEAVES

Urinary system

Women are vulnerable to urinary infections (because of their short urethra); men are more at risk of kidney stones. Many essential oils are relaxing, diuretic, pain-relieving, and anti-inflammatory.

KIDNEY STONES

Minerals in urine can crystallize into stones in the kidneys and bladder, causing severe pain. Geranium, juniper, lemon, or fennel oil can be used in the bath or massaged into the bladder area.

CYSTITIS

An infected urethra or bladder causes frequent, painful urination and abdominal pain. Suitable oils include bergamot, cedarwood, eucalyptus, frankincense, juniper, lavender, sandalwood, tea tree, camomile, pine, and angelica: add to bathwater or use in a compress.

THRUSH

Overgrowth of this yeastlike micro-organism leads to infection. Tea tree oil has powerful antifungal and antiseptic properties. Other oils include lavender, juniper, myrrh, and sandalwood: add to the bath.

URETHRITIS

An inflamed and infected urethra may cause a sore penis in men, painful urination, and possibly discharge. Bergamot, lavender, and sandalwood are antiseptic and pain-relieving: add to bathwater.

Many essential oils help urinary infections in women.

URINARY SYSTEM

The urinary system deals with the elimination of excess water and waste products.

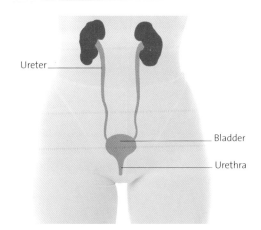

Ureter — Bladder — Urethra

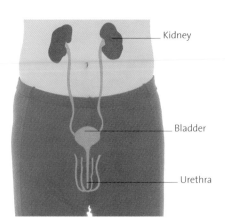

Kidney — Bladder — Urethra

Men have fewer problems with infection and urinary control because the urethra is five times longer than in women.

Reproductive system

Certain essential oils have an affinity with the reproductive system and may regulate hormonal imbalances.

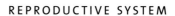

CLARY
SAGE

PREMENSTRUAL SYNDROME (PMS)

Alleviate water retention and irritability with rosemary, cypress, or patchouli oils added to bathwater. Massage with lavender, geranium, frankincense, or sandalwood for relaxation; rose, jasmine, and clary sage to improve mood.

PERIOD PROBLEMS

Treat heavy bleeding with yarrow, lemon, geranium, hyssop, rose, or cypress added to the bath or used as a massage oil. Ease period pains with clary sage, marjoram, vetiver, peppermint, lavender, or cypress.

INFERTILITY

Try rosemary, geranium, and lavender to relieve stress and tension. Peppermint and ginger act as a general tonic. Rose and melissa are thought to have a particular affinity with the reproductive organs.

LOSS OF LIBIDO AND IMPOTENCE

Many essential oils are natural aphrodisiacs. Try a massage or bath with sandalwood, jasmine, rose, ylang ylang, or rosemary. Lavender, marjoram, myrtle, geranium, and bergamot are beneficial for sexual problems caused by stress.

REPRODUCTIVE SYSTEM

Male and female reproductive systems comprise organs for sexual intercourse and reproduction. They are aided by essential oils.

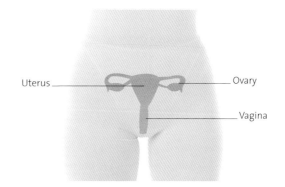

Uterus — Ovary

Vagina

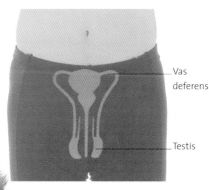

Vas deferens

Testis

Essential oils can alienate a number of conditions that affect fertility and sexual function.

Essential oils have long been used to treat problems of libido and impotence.

LAVENDER

Special cases

Essential oils are particularly appropriate at certain times of life: during childhood, for women during pregnancy and the menopause, and in old age.

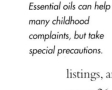

Essential oils can help many childhood complaints, but take special precautions.

CHILDHOOD

Do not use oils in the bath or on the skin until a child is at least a year old. Alleviate sleep problems by adding a few drops of camomile, lavender, rose, or geranium to the bathwater, or give a gentle massage with lavender or camomile in a carrier oil before bedtime, or use in a vaporizer. Lavender, rose, camomile, sandalwood, and neroli can be used in a massage or added to the bath to calm a hyperactive child.

PREGNANCY

A range of complaints may arise during pregnancy, including hemorrhoids, constipation, fluid retention, backache, insomnia, and morning sickness. See previous listings, and check the information for each oil on pages 26–73 to ensure it is safe to use during pregnancy. Avoid massage and use the oils in a vaporizer until the fifth month of pregnancy. Lavender, camomile, and marjoram ease muscular pains. Massage neroli, palmarosa, mandarin, or lavender into the abdominal region to help prevent stretch marks.

CHILDBIRTH

Certain oils may be used when labor is established to hasten contractions, notably jasmine, clove, rose, and clary sage. Camomile, rubbed into the abdominal region, relieves pain. Melissa and lavender can be used throughout labor.

POST-DELIVERY PROBLEMS

Geranium, clary sage, and rose are uterine tonics and help the pelvic muscles regain their elasticity. Lavender and camomile can be applied diluted to painful stitches. Fennel or lemongrass compresses may stimulate breast milk flow.

POSTNATAL ILLNESS

Jasmine, bergamot, ylang ylang, neroli, lavender, and clary sage can be added to the bath or used in a massage to balance hormones, relax the body, and ease symptoms.

MENOPAUSE

Camomile, fennel, and clary sage help to balance hormone levels. Geranium, jasmine, and ylang ylang are appropriate for low libido.

THE ELDERLY

Essential oils can be used throughout life, but elderly people may prefer to have a hand, foot, or face massage rather than a full body massage.

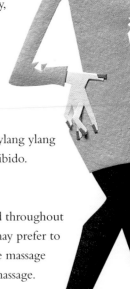

Camomile, fennel, and clary sage help to balance hormonel levels.

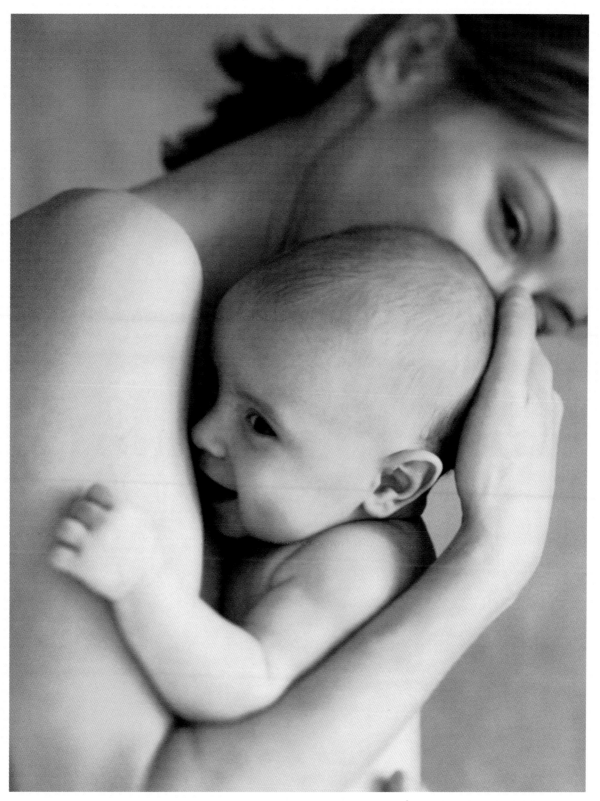

*Many essential oils can help both before
and after pregnancy.*

First **aid**

Essential oils can bring instant relief in many first-aid situations. Seek medical advice if the person affected has a high temperature or has a severe allergic reaction.

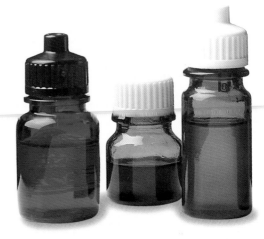

A few bottles of essential oils are useful additions to a first-aid box.

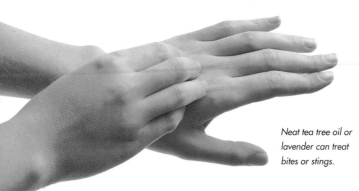

Neat tea tree oil or lavender can treat bites or stings.

BITES AND STINGS

Itching and inflammation may be relieved by the antiseptic and anti-inflammatory action of several oils. Use a drop of neat lavender or tea tree oil to treat bites or stings. Geranium, melissa, basil, and fennel can be used in a compress or in the bath.

BRUISES

Dab neat lavender or geranium oil on to a bruise. Other oils can be used in a cold compress: clary sage, angelica, rosemary, fennel, marjoram, cypress, and ginger are suitable.

BURNS

Mild burns and scalds respond well to essential oils. Flood the area with cold water first or apply a cold compress. A drop of tea tree oil or lavender can be used neat immediately after the accident. Geranium, eucalyptus, rose, and camomile are soothing and healing.

SUNBURN

Treat sunburn as you would any other burn. The oils listed can be added to bathwater or used in lotions or a cool compress: cypress, cedarwood, eucalyptus, geranium, jasmine, lavender, neroli, patchouli rose, sandalwood, and tea tree.

Add cypress, cedarwood, eucalyptus, geranium, or jasmine oil to body lotion to help treat sunburn.

ALLERGIC REACTIONS

An allergy is an abnormal response of the immune system to a specific substance, and manifests as sneezing, urticaria (hives), breathing difficulties, and anaphylactic shock in serious cases, which can be fatal. Essential oils are very effective in reducing spasms and the severity of the reaction. Massage lavender oil into the chest area. Soothing camomile, lavender, and melissa can be added to bathwater or used in a vaporizer.

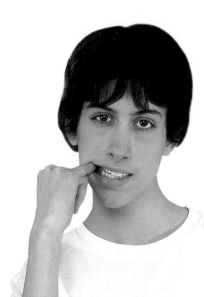

Peppermint and clove oil rubbed directly on the tooth can temporarily ease toothache.

FAINTING

Massage rosemary into the temples to prevent fainting episodes. A drop of peppermint oil or neroli on a handkerchief may revive senses when you feel faint, or in cases of shock.

PEPPERMINT

TOOTHACHE

Apply a drop of peppermint or clove oil directly to the tooth for pain relief. Rub lavender on the jaw and face to ease pain and discomfort.

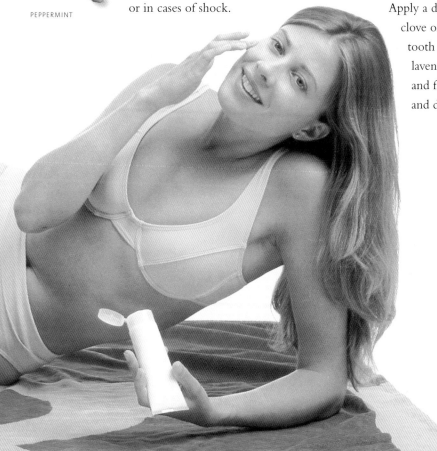

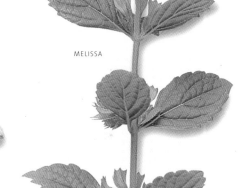

MELISSA

Glossary

ACUTE a disorder of sudden onset

ANALGESIC relieves pain

ANTI-INFLAMMATORY reduces inflammation

ANTIDEPRESSANT uplifting

ANTI-FUNGAL reduces fungal growth

ANTISEPTIC reduces bacterial growth

ANTISPASMODIC reduces muscle spasms and cramps

ANTIVIRAL controls viruses

APERITIF stimulates appetite

APHRODISIAC increases sexual desire

ASTRINGENT drying, contracts body tissues

BACTERICIDAL combats bacteria

CARMINATIVE relaxes the stomach and relieves flatulence

CHRONIC a condition of long duration and slow changes

CICATRISANT promotes the formation of scar tissue

DECONGESTANT relieves the accumulation of mucus

DEODORIZING prevents body odour

DETOXIFY purge poisons and waste products produced by the body

DIGESTIVE aids digestion

DISINFECTANT destroys germs

DIURETIC promotes urination

EMOLLIENT soothes and softens the skin

EXPECTORANT expels mucus from the lungs

FEBRIFUGAL lowers temperature and relieves fever

GERMICIDAL kills germs and bacteria

INSECTICIDAL kills insects

LAXATIVE promotes bowel action

PHOTOTOXIC increases the skin's sensitivity to sunlight

RELAXANT relieves tension

RUBEFACIENT reddens the skin and increases circulation

SEDATIVE calms the nerves

STIMULANT increases activity

TONIC strengthens a system or organ

UTERINE for the uterus

Useful addresses

Further information available from:

American Alliance of Aromatherapy
P.O. Box 750428
Petaluma
CA 94975-0428

American Aromatherapy Association
P.O. Box 3679
South Pasadena
CA 91031

National Association for Holistic Aromatherapy
P.O. Box 17622
Boulder
CO 80308-0622

National Association for Holistic Aromatherapy (NAHA)
4509 Interlake Ave N 233
Seattle
WA 981093-2680
www.naha.org

Real Essences Aromatherapy
2122b MacDonald Street
Vancouver
British Columbia
V6K 3Y4
Canada

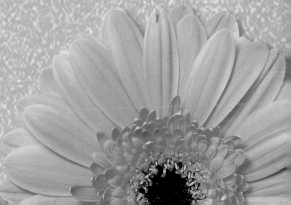

Index

Acknowledgements

Special thanks go to
Jane Lanaway for design and
photography co-ordination
Malika Hopkins, Stephanie Winter
and Ian Parsons for help
with photography

*The publishers would like to thank
the following for the use of pictures:*
Corbis 8/9, 10, 10/11, 21, 31,
35, 38, 45, 51, 54, 55, 62,
67, 69, 78/79
Harry Smith Collection 46
Image Bank 15. 56
Images Colour Library
26/27, 42
Stone Gettyone 1, 7, 32, 37,
64, 74/75, 76/77, 91
Superstock 13
The Garden Picture Library 39
Vanessa Fletcher 28, 43
Trudi Valter for
picture research